THE
Buena Salud™
GUIDE
FOR A
HEALTHY
HEART

Newmarket Books by Jane L. Delgado, Ph.D., M.S.

The Buena Salud™ Guide for a Healthy Heart

The Buena Salud™ Guide to Diabetes and Your Life

The Latina Guide to Health: Consejos and Caring Answers

[all available in English and Spanish]

THE
Buena Salud™
GUIDE
FOR A
HEALTHY
HEART

JANE L. DELGADO, PH.D., M.S.

Foreword by John C. Lewin, M.D.
CEO, American College of Cardiology, Washington, D.C.

NEWMARKET PRESS

This book is published in the United States of America.

First Edition

ISBN: 978-1-55704-943-8 (English-language paperback)
1 2 3 4 5 6 7 8 9 10

ISBN: 978-1-55704-944-5 (Spanish-language paperback)
1 2 3 4 5 6 7 8 9 10

Library of Congress Cataloging-in-Publication Data

Delgado, Jane L.
  The buena salud™ guide for a healthy heart / Jane L. Delgado; foreword by John C. Lewin. -- 1st ed.
     p. cm.
  Includes index.
  Published simultaneously in Spanish under the title: La guia de Buena Salud™ para un corazon sano.
   ISBN 978-1-55704-943-8
  1. Heart--Diseases--Popular works. 2. Hispanic Americans--Health and hygiene--Popular works. I. Title.
   RC672.D45 2011
   616.1'208968'073--dc22
                          2010041609

QUANTITY PURCHASES
Companies, professional groups, clubs, and other organizations may qualify for special terms when ordering quantities of this title. For information e-mail sales@newmarketpress.com or write to Special Sales Department, Newmarket Press, 18 East 48th Street, New York, NY 10017; call (212) 832-3575 ext. 19 or 1-800-669-3903; FAX (212) 832-3629.

Web site: www.newmarketpress.com

Design by Keira McGuinness

Manufactured in the United States of America.

⌒ Contents

CONTENTS

PART TWO: JUST THE FACTS *(continued)*

You say I have . . .

Diagnostic Tests and Procedures

PART TWO: JUST THE FACTS (*continued*)

**PART THREE: RESOURCES AND TOOLS
TO HELP YOU TAKE CONTROL**

The *Buena Salud*™ Series

The mission of the National Alliance for Hispanic Health (the Alliance) is to improve the health of Hispanic communities and work with others to secure health for all. This has been a major challenge because although 1 out of every 6 people in the United States is Hispanic, too often the research, analysis, and recommendations do not address Hispanic lives. As information emerges about Hispanic health, it is clear that to achieve the best health outcomes for all, we need a different approach to health care in our communities. Besides providing the best health information, we need to create a new way to think about health that blends the strengths of the Hispanic community with the latest medical and technological advances.

The *Buena Salud*™ series is designed to make that happen. Each book identifies the key factors that define a health concern, the changes that each of us needs to consider making for ourselves and our family, the most up-to-date information to live healthier lives, and the tools that we need to make that possible.

The challenge is to sort through the daily onslaught of health-related information and recognize that many of the changes we need to make to improve our health we cannot do alone. Our sense of family and responsibility to our family is one of the great strengths in our community, and it is key to improving the health system. Nevertheless, to do so we all need to work together. Whether it is an uncle, a brother, a sister, or a *comadre*, we have to help each other

9

become as healthy as possible. This series is for you because there is so much that you can do to improve your own health and the health of others.

We are at a critical moment when we can make all of our lives better. The promise of science is before us, and we must use every bit of information to care for our body, mind, and spirit. Through the *Buena Salud*™ series, we want to be your partner in making it happen.

⌒Foreword

Those of you who do not personally have the pleasure of knowing Dr. Jane Delgado, chief executive of the National Alliance for Hispanic Health, have not yet fully lived. She is one of the few Washington, D.C., association leaders with compassion, common sense, and an uncanny ability to bring people and diverse groups together to solve problems. She is also an accomplished author and educator. In writing this new and timely book, *The Buena Salud™ Guide for a Healthy Heart*, Dr. Delgado opens windows to her unique and refreshingly clear views on cardiovascular health and health care, and shows why you should pay attention to what she has learned in these regards.

Her "10-Point Program for Health" combines both common sense and what you might have been once taught by your grandmother. Most of us have apparently forgotten to apply much of this sound advice in our own lives.

Dr. Delgado applies to your potential well-being what the best clinical science tells us about cardiovascular disease and health. She highlights what we know about current medical treatment options and prevention advice and strategies, along with offering some important resources to help us take control of our own health and/or to help our loved ones to do so.

The author also demystifies, in laypeople's terms, many of the complicated cardiovascular diagnoses and the technologies and tests used to discover and treat heart disease. Medical terminology and technology can confuse or overwhelm people without a medical background who have or are at risk of heart disease. Dr. Delgado makes all of this easier to understand and consider.

Everybody needs this kind of information. But, as many of us as physicians have learned, the CHO (chief health officer) of the family is statistically most often a woman—a wife, a mother, or a sister. Women are far more likely than the "less aware gender" to take charge of helping members of the immediate and extended *familia* to exercise personal responsibility for their health, whether it's exercising, eating well, getting enough sleep, or cherishing their spiritual life.

Dr. Delgado understands the importance of family and community in promoting healthier behaviors, and she presents ways to do so that are practical and realistic for families of all kinds. CHOs of families everywhere, whether Hispanic or not, will find this information—and Dr. Delgado's easily understandable way of communicating it—invaluable in helping to manage both their own cardiovascular health and that of those they love.

This good advice is also particularly pertinent for men and women. There are major differences between the sexes, as well as differences between members of various ethnic and cultural groups, when it comes to cardiovascular disease and risk, symptomatology, and best-care strategies. Heart disease is the number-one cause of morbidity (illness) and mortality worldwide, even in China, India, and South and Central America. And since the mid-1980s, more women than men have died of cardiovascular disease, a fact that too many patients and doctors seem not to recognize.

Dr. Delgado understands! She recognizes the need to approach health care according to individual, ethnic, cultural, and religious differences and preferences if we want to be effective. Personalizing care requires knowing as much as possible about what the scientific facts and clinical options are. That's why you need to read this book and share it with your family and friends. We all need to better understand how to take greater responsibility for our own personal and family health. We need to be able to identify cardiovascular risks early and avoid larger problems in the future.

I enthusiastically recommend *The Buena Salud™ Guide for a Healthy Heart*. Read it. Recommend it. Most important, use it to make a real difference in improving your own heart health and to contribute to a needed revolution in prevention, improved chronic disease management, and personal health responsibility.

—JOHN C. (JACK) LEWIN, MD
CEO, AMERICAN COLLEGE OF CARDIOLOGY
WASHINGTON, D.C.

⌒Introduction

I t has taken me seventeen years since my mother died from heart disease to be able to write extensively about this topic. All my research has documented that the amount of progress that has been made in this short time is not only amazing, but it could have saved my mother's life. Today both men and women are more likely to survive bypass surgery than they were in the past. Moreover, fewer of us need bypass surgery, as the variety of medications and minimally invasive procedures that are available to resolve and control heart and related problems make bypass surgery less necessary.

Too often we use the term *heart disease* to cover everything from problems with how our heart actually works to problems with our blood vessels. *Heart disease* is the more popular way to refer to cardiovascular disease. By presenting information in this book in a manner that includes the experiences of real people, it is my hope that you will be able to take steps to develop and maintain the healthiest heart possible.

I want you and all those you care for to have the most up-to-date facts; explanations of the more common conditions, diagnostic tools, and procedures; tools to help you monitor your own health; and resources that you can trust.

The key factor to recognize about heart disease and related conditions is that your heart is not just a pump. If you think of your heart as nothing more than a pump, you miss that the heart is part of your circulatory system, electrical system, and a system that is connected to your thoughts and feelings. These facts will help you understand the actions you can take to make it all work well and give you the robust health you want.

Part One

MORE THAN YOUR HEART

What do we really know about the heart and Hispanics?

I know when my mother's heart condition really began. It was when she heard the news that her sister had died. My mother had survived all sorts of hardship with the hope and dream that, when she was older, she and her sister would finally be able to live together and enjoy life. Those were the plans that mom and *Tía* made. And when life was tough it was the vision of the two of them living the last years of their lives together that sustained my mother.

I was at work when my mother received the news that her sister had died. When I got home that evening, Mom told me what had happened. She did not cry, as that was not her way. All I saw in her eyes and on her face was that her spirit had been crushed.

My mother had always been a vibrant and energetic woman, but somehow, with the news of *Tía's* death, everything changed. Her smile became a motion she did with her lips, as her eyes lost their sparkle and brightness.

A few months later she had the first of a series of heart attacks and had to start seeing a cardiologist. It surprised many of her friends that she would have heart disease; after all, she was not overweight, she

exercised nearly every day of her life, and she walked
on a regular basis. Only I saw the depth of her sadness.
And because I recognized how profoundly her sadness
affected her soul, I witnessed what happened. I saw
how a heart can be broken by a sadness that is incon-
solable because there is no hope.

Heart disease is the number-one cause of death for all of us—Hispanics, non-Hispanics, Latinos, and Latinas. It is so common to have a condition related to the heart that most of us know someone who is either taking medicines to avoid having a heart problem or doing something to develop a healthier heart. And while you may have some knowledge about the heart and how it works, the facts need to be analyzed using a different lens when someone is Hispanic.

For many years, when researchers did studies on the heart, most of what they knew was based on research on non-Hispanic white men. The belief was that all people were the same. Eventually, data were collected on African Americans and women. As these data were deciphered, it became clear that there were differences among the groups. Nevertheless, the tendency was to apply what was known about African Americans to explain the health of Hispanics. At the time, researchers believed that all minorities would have the same health issues.

By 1990, the government started to collect data on the cause of death for Hispanics. The early results were confusing. It seemed that, while heart disease was the number-one cause of death for Hispanic men and women, the disease unfolded in ways that were different from how it proceeded among other racial and ethnic groups. It was becoming increasingly clear that the risk factors for heart disease that were so prevalent in the Hispanic community did not result in a corresponding increase in heart disease.

Specifically, when compared to non-Hispanic whites, Hispanics were more likely to carry excess weight and more likely to have type 2 diabetes. This was true for both Hispanic men and Hispanic women. What was different is that, even though Hispanics had these major risk factors, they did not seem to result in the higher rates of heart disease that would have been predicted by existing models.

This unusual finding was initially either ignored or explained away as the result of bad data collection. As the years passed, the consistency with which this finding occurred, across states and regardless of specific country of origin, made researchers curious as to what was going on.

These differences were discovered at about the same time that we were gaining a deeper understanding of the human genome. Research needed to be done to understand why Hispanics were experiencing heart disease in ways that did not follow the recognized models.

Soon it became clear that whatever was going on did not involve a genetic difference, because the health advantage diminished over time. The difference had to do with how we lived our lives. Ironically, those of us who were in the United States longer seemed to lose the health benefits that our parents enjoyed. The more we adapted to and adopted the U.S. lifestyle, the worse our health became. This finding is consistent across many immigrant groups.

That the first immigrant groups have better health outcomes than those of us who have been here for generations should come as no surprise. We are humans, and when humans have more options, we do not necessarily make the best choices.

Consequently, what the data show are that, over time, immigrants start to smoke, they drive rather than walk, they drink more alcohol, they eat foods that are fast to prepare, and they become more ruggedly individualistic rather than maintaining a family or community orientation.

These factors, and the understanding of how they work, are so critical that the National Heart, Lung, and Blood Institute (NHLBI), a division of the National Institutes of Health (NIH), is undertaking a major study of 16,000 Hispanics across the nation (in San Diego, Chicago, New York, and Miami) to unravel the factors that lead to the Hispanic portrait of heart disease. Most of the findings from these studies will not be available for several years. That is why it is not surprising that our knowledge about the heart and heart-related diseases among Hispanics is often not as accurate as it could be.

How the heart works

A healthy adult heart is a muscular organ, about the size of a person's fist, and it is located in the middle of the chest. The inside of the heart has four parts, called chambers (the upper two are called atria; the lower two are called ventricles), a wall that separates the left from the right side of the heart (the septum), and four valves (the aortic valve, the tricuspid valve, the pulmonary valve, and the mitral valve). The outside of the heart is connected to some major arteries (coronary arteries) and veins (the superior and inferior vena cava).

Your heart beats about 100,000 times a day. With every beat, the heart pumps blood to every cell in the body and takes away the waste products that are produced by our cells and tissues. The blood travels in one direction through the arteries, veins, capillaries, and blood vessels, and then back to the lungs. These different types of blood vessels (arterial, venous, capillary, and pulmonary) make up the circulatory system. Now, as you take your next breath, try to understand how intricate this all is.

Think of what happens each time your heart beats. The electrical signals and valves in your heart work in unison to pump blood rich in oxygen to your arteries. Healthy arteries that are flexible and muscular accommodate the changes that are needed to transport blood to every part of your body through a network of blood vessels of varying sizes. The arteries have offshoots that are smaller blood vessels, called arterioles, which lead to the even smaller capillaries, which bring the oxygen-rich blood to your organs and tissue. Capillaries, with their dual action, then connect to your veins. Veins carry blood that does not have oxygen back to the lungs in order to get replenished with fresh oxygen. Then the heart beats again and the cycle repeats itself. Depending on the needs of the body, and how much you are exerting yourself, your heartbeat may be faster or slower.

All this occurs in a matter of seconds and is possible because the heart is part of many systems—circulatory, electrical, and even a system that is mediated by your thoughts and feelings.

CIRCULATORY SYSTEM

THIS SYSTEM IS MADE UP OF YOUR HEART AND FOUR DIFFERENT TYPES of systems that move blood in different directions in your body.

The *arterial circulation system* focuses on arteries. Arteries help move blood away from the heart and are strong and elastic. Healthy arteries are key to having normal blood pressure.

The *venous circulation system* involves the blood vessels that bring blood to the heart. The walls of veins are thinner than the walls of arteries, and have the capacity to widen to transport more blood.

The *capillary circulation system* is made up of very small blood vessels, called capillaries. Capillaries are the thinnest blood vessels of all, and are specialized to connect to both arteries and veins. Their thin walls make it possible to transport both nutrients and oxygen and take away the carbon dioxide that is produced as waste by organs and tissues in the body.

The *pulmonary circulation system* deals with the heart and lungs working together. Arteries, veins, and capillaries make it possible to transport blood without oxygen from the heart to the lungs and blood with oxygen from the lungs back to the heart.

ELECTRICAL SYSTEM

EACH HEARTBEAT BEGINS IN THE UPPER RIGHT CHAMBER OF THE heart, where special cells give off an electrical signal. The electrical signal is what makes the heart contract and pump blood as it travels from the top of the heart to the bottom. In a healthy heart, the signal travels in a set path. It makes the upper chambers contract and pump blood to both lower chambers, then slows down for an instant to allow the lower chambers of the heart to fill with blood. Then the electrical current continues its journey to pump blood out from both sides of the lower chambers. The electrical signal to contract goes to both lower chambers. The lower-left chamber (the ventricle), which pushes the blood throughout your body, contracts an instant before the lower-right chamber, which pushes the blood to the lungs. Once the signal has completed its journey through the heart, the walls of the lower chamber of your heart relax and get ready for the next signal. This electrical signal occurs 60 to 100 times per minute throughout your adult life.

THOUGHTS AND FEELINGS

THOUGHTS AND FEELINGS DEFINITELY IMPACT OUR HEART. But how that connection works is what we know the least about, when it comes to the heart. The data clearly link depression and heart disease. This is important for Hispanics, as we are more likely to suffer from untreated depression than non-Hispanic whites.

Researchers are not certain as to which came first—the depression or the heart problem. What we do know is that those with depression are more likely to have a heart problem than those who are not depressed. For women, the relationship between depression and heart problems seems more immediate. For men, it is more difficult to untangle, because too often mainstream society encourages men to ignore what they feel and just get done whatever has to get done.

Our feelings are real and, whether we acknowledge them or not, they have a major influence on our physical health. And our heart is very much affected by the people and experiences that frame our daily life. It seems as if the disavowing of feelings puts men at greater risk of heart problems than women. Men with feelings of hostility and internalized anger are more likely to develop heart problems. While scientists may still be seeking answers to the nature of that connection, the fact is that it definitely exists.

Just as certain is the negative impact that stress has on our heart. That is why, for women, we know that stress results in increased production of the hormone cortisol that is produced by the adrenal glands. The cortisol response tends to make women accumulate more belly fat, and belly fat puts a person at increased risk for heart disease. It is still not known why this response does not occur in men. The issue may be related to how women handle stress as compared to men.

We all know stress and feel stress, and yet how we respond to stress varies by individual and situation. We only have to look at our relationships with others to know that men and women handle stress in different ways. Broadly speaking, researchers have documented that when men experience stress, their reactions fall along the continuum of fight or flight. In the fight response, the person prepares for combat, becomes aggressive, and confronts the situation. In the flight response, the person tries to get away from, or flee, the situation. This includes withdrawing from people, abusing alcohol or other substances, or even engaging in excessive television viewing.

For too long we used this theory to explain how everyone handled stress. We ignored that people sometimes respond to stressful situations by joining with others to provide mutual protection. More recently, with research on how women handle stress, another series of responses have emerged. It seems that, in stressful situations, women initiate a "tend" (taking care of children and others) and "befriend" (talking to others) response.

Although this idea that men and women handle stress differently is useful, it does not capture the vitality that makes each one of us respond in a different and somewhat distinctive way. To a certain degree, our responses to stress all fall somewhere along the fight-or-flight and the tend-and-befriend continuums, depending on the situation. If someone with a weapon is chasing us, we may all engage in a "flight" response. Our response is not as clear when the stress is created by not knowing how to handle someone we love who is becoming increasingly difficult to live with. The key concern here is this:

Depending on how much personal emotional stress you feel, that stress will produce a different impact on your heart. And too much stress is not good for the heart.

Understanding how the heart works makes it clear that there is no single action that will ensure a healthy heart. Not only are there too many factors to consider, but also there are factors that are simply beyond our control. Moreover, there is a lot of distance between what we can and should do. The challenge is to take as many positive actions for you and your family without creating more stress in your life.

Life changes to consider: Things to do and things to avoid

Heart disease rarely develops suddenly. In most cases, it is a process that evolves over time. To have a healthy heart we need to make changes in our lifestyle. This is difficult even when those changes are for our own good. It is not that we want to make choices that are not good for us, but rather that it takes an effort to do what is good for us. No one strives for bad health; we just seem to get there over time. We do not wake up one morning and say to ourselves, "Look what happened overnight." It is our everyday decisions and habits that we have to reconsider.

It takes sustained effort to do what is good for us because contemporary life makes it easier to make bad choices. It is amazing to me that health care professionals believe that just giving someone information is enough to prompt them to change their behavior. We should all know better. Ask any one of us and we can tell you what steps we need to take to have a healthy heart. But knowledge and information are not enough.

What I want you to do is to take what you already know, add to that the new science I share with you, and try to reconsider the things that you can do. Look at the questions below and answer each one.

- Do you stay away from smoke and toxic air? ☐ yes ☐ no
- In addition to your regular routine, do you try to keep moving? ☐ yes ☐ no
- Do you eat for a healthy heart? ☐ yes ☐ no
- Do you get enough sleep? ☐ yes ☐ no
- Do you have healthy relationships? ☐ yes ☐ no
- Do you have a regular source of health care? ☐ yes ☐ no
- Do you keep a journal of your health? ☐ yes ☐ no
- Do you cherish your spiritual life? ☐ yes ☐ no
- Do you take your medications as prescribed? ☐ yes ☐ no
- Do you know how to listen to your body? ☐ yes ☐ no

Now look at your answers. For each question to which you answered "no," read the sections below, choose 3 that you will work on, and make a decision to take the necessary steps to move your life in a heart-healthier direction. Then read the sections where you answered "yes" and use the information to reaffirm the heart-healthful steps you are already taking.

10-POINT PROGRAM FOR HEALTH

1. STAY AWAY FROM SMOKE AND TOXIC AIR

EVERY TIME YOU BREATHE IN, YOUR LUNGS AND HEART WORK together to fill the cells that do not have oxygen with the air you just took in. The oxygen-filled cells then travel throughout your body to every tissue and organ. If the air you breathe in is toxic, then that is what will fill the cells in your body.

Tobacco is an air pollutant, and it is toxic. Decades of research make it clear that smoking is bad for people who smoke, those who are near them when they smoke (secondhand smoke), and even the people who only inhale the lingering smell of tobacco that clings to a smoker's clothes and hair (thirdhand smoke). It is getting easier to stay away from smoke, as more and more places are banning smoking.

That is why, during days when the air quality is poor, if you go outside and breathe the air, you are more likely to end up in the emergency room with a heart problem. The federal Environmental Protection Agency (EPA) is starting to tighten many of the restrictions on the levels of pollutants in the air. We already know that there are too many pollutants and toxic substances and that the EPA keeps track of very few of them. Some airborne toxins include benzene (which is found in gasoline), dioxin, asbestos, toluene, and metals, such as cadmium, mercury, chromium, and lead compounds.

Keep in mind that sometimes the most hazardous particles to breathe in are the ones that you cannot see. According to the EPA, the air contains "inhalable coarse particles" (PM_{10}, or between 2.5 and 10 micrometers in diameter) as well as "fine particles" ($PM_{2.5}$, or less than 2.5 micrometers in diameter). It takes at least 28 fine particles to be as wide as a strand of hair. The fine particles are more dangerous to our health because they settle more deeply in our lungs.

While the air outside is a problem, the air inside can be a problem, too. Many products give off gases that are called volatile organic compounds (VOCs), some of which may have short- and/or long-term adverse health effects. Household products that usually release VOCs include paints, paint strippers and thinners, and other solvents; wood preservatives; aerosol sprays; cleansers and disinfectants; moth repellents; air fresheners; stored fuels and automotive products; hobby supplies such as airplane glue; and clothing dry-cleaned with perchlorethlyene. That smell of fresh paint or new carpeting is not good for your health. And some dangerous indoor substances, like radon, have no smell at all; they can only be detected with special equipment.

2. KEEP MOVING

For as long as I have been married to Juan, he does the same thing every day. He wakes up every morning and goes on his exercise bicycle for sixty minutes. If you looked at him, you wouldn't know it because he does not look like someone who exercises. I don't understand that. —Rebecca

I spend my day working, working, working. When I get home I just want to relax and do nothing. I am too tired to exercise. Just making dinner is an effort for me. At the end of the day, I have no energy... there is nothing left. —Jeannie

FOR MANY OF US, THE DAILY ROUTINE IS PHYSICALLY EXHAUSTING and leaves us too tired to think of much else. Research confirms that most of us have to increase our physical activity in ways that are good for our heart. Some people may want to dance or run a marathon and will do so. Most of us will have to find activities that we can do on a consistent basis for the rest of our lives.

The key word here is *activities,* in the plural. If we do the same activity at the same time every day, our body, being the wonderful adaptive machine that it is, gets accustomed to whatever we are doing and we do not seem to get as much benefit from that activity. Our challenge is to find what variety of activities will work for us.

This is actually very difficult to do because it demands that we put out energy when we really may want to rest. But to have a healthy heart, we have to get up and do something.

The best kind of physical activity is the one you will do on a consistent basis. While your heart demands that you build your heart muscle through aerobic activities, to maintain your overall health you also have to exercise to strengthen your muscles and bones as well as stretch to maintain your flexibility.

When you do aerobic activities, your heart beats more and you breathe harder than usual. The more you do these activities, the stronger your heart and lungs become. Muscle strengthening is about making all your muscles (in your legs, hips, back, chest, abdomen, shoulders, and arms) stronger by lifting weights, digging in the garden, working with resistance bands, or doing sit-ups. Since your bones are alive, you need to strengthen them, too. Bone-strengthening exercises are whatever make your feet, legs, or arms support the full weight of your body. These activities make your muscles push against your bones; for example, dancing, walking, jumping rope, or lifting weights. Stretching is key to flexibility and the ability to move your muscles without injury. Mix it up and do what you can. It helps to keep a written record of what you do so that you can see the progress that you have made—or failed to make.

The goal is simple. You have to keep your whole body moving as much as possible. Moderation is key to continuing to do whatever you do. While there is a place for extreme sports, such activities are not part of a long-term health strategy that you will be able to maintain for the rest of your life.

But how intense does exercise have to be? It all depends on you and your level of heart health and overall fitness. In general, if you are walking, you should be able to talk and walk at the same time. If you are out of breath and cannot speak, then you are walking too fast or on too difficult a course.

Do as much as you can whenever you can. Even 10-minute bursts of exercise 3 times a day several days a week is better than nothing. There are so many benefits to being physically active. You just have to keep doing whatever you do.

Highlights of Recommendations for Physical Activity
In 2008 the U.S. Department of Health and Human Services released new physical activity guidelines. Ask your health care provider which activities are safe for you. If you are inactive, you should gradually increase your activity level and not begin with vigorous activity. Even if you played some sport when you were younger, you have to ease back into it if you have not done it for a while. For adults, the guidelines advise that:

- Something is better than nothing. If you are just starting an exercise program, you should gradually increase your level of activity. As little as 60 minutes of moderate-intensity aerobic activity per week is beneficial.

- For major health benefits, do at least 150 minutes of moderate-intensity aerobic activity or 75 minutes of vigorous-intensity aerobic activity each week. The more you do, the greater the benefits to your heart.

- Do aerobic activities for at least 10 minutes at a time several times a week.

- Muscle-strengthening activities that are moderate or high intensity should be included 2 or more days a week.

- Be as physically active as your abilities and condition allow, because any amount of physical activity will produce some health benefits.

3. EAT AND DRINK FOR A HEALTHY HEART

THE FIRST PLACE TO START IS TO ELIMINATE THE WORD *DIET* FROM your vocabulary. Instead, what you eat will be driven by your new goal to eat for a healthy heart, based on the latest research. This is a good thing for everyone to do, since it will make you and your family healthier. What is good for your heart is also good for your overall health and mood.

I know that I do not have to go into detail about what is good for you and what you should eat only rarely. Your new way to eat will focus on the 3 principles of healthy eating: pleasure, portion, and process.

Pleasure

You have to think about what you are eating. It means that you cannot sit and mindlessly eat. You cannot inhale your food. You cannot eat just because the bell goes off and it is noon. You have to eat to enjoy what you eat and the full experience of eating, preferably with others. This means you should eat slowly and never talk with your mouth full. It means thinking about what you eat and what it does for your heart. As the food goes into your mouth, it is to satisfy your taste buds. Eating is about the pleasure of indulging in different flavors and the pleasant memories that the aromas evoke. It is not about stuffing yourself. We have to think about eating in a new way. A buffet is not a challenge to see how high you can pile up food on one plate, but instead a sumptuous array of different flavors you can savor. Drinking red wine (one glass is 5 ounces) for pleasure and your health means no more than two glasses a day for healthy men up to age 65 and no more than one glass a day for healthy women and healthy men over age 65.

Portion
Servings should not be one size fits all. This means that our portions need to match our rate of metabolism. Athletes or younger people may have larger portions because their bodies use the food more quickly than those who are less active. As we get older, the portion that we need gets smaller.

Process
How did the food get to your plate? The less processing involved, the better. You have to read the food label to know what is in the food you buy. This means eliminating from your eating plan foods with trans fats; avoiding sodium; and consuming only minimal amounts of chemicals or preservatives. There are so many tasty choices to enjoy: beans, brown rice, breads and pasta that are made with whole grains, fresh fruits rather than juice or juice drinks, plantains, fresh or frozen vegetables, meat that is not processed, water instead of energy drinks, fish that is sustainable, nuts, and so much more. If you want to sweeten your food, think raw sugar or agave instead of white sugar. The principle is simple: Enjoy more of what is less processed.

Finally, if you think about what you eat and how your body uses what you consume, you will be able to make better choices. As an added plus, you will be more comfortable when you do physical activities.

4. GET ENOUGH SLEEP

YOU NEED TO GET SLEEP. SLEEP IS DIFFERENT THAN REST OR DOING nothing. Sleep is a function that your body needs to stay healthy. If you have a sleep disorder, you are at a higher risk of high blood pressure, heart attack, stroke, and other medical conditions.

When you sleep, your heart rate and blood pressure go down about 10 percent. People who do not get enough sleep do not have this reduction and compromise the health of their heart. When you do not sleep, your body is under stress and that changes the hormones your body produces. This increases your risk of heart disease.

The hormones that are released when you sleep are very important. Besides making you more alert, the hormones that control your appetite are also activated while you sleep. People who sleep only 5 hours a night are more likely to have excess weight than those who sleep 7 to 8 hours per night.

How much sleep you need varies by age: Healthy adults need 7 to 9 hours of sleep, newborns 16 to 18 hours, children in preschool 10 to 12 hours, and school-aged children and adolescents at least 9 hours. No wonder it is so hard to get everybody in the house moving at the same time. But quality of sleep is as important as quantity. Short (less than 1-hour) daytime naps can only partially make up for missed sleep. Keep in mind that you cannot make up for sleep lost during the week by sleeping more on the weekends, and this type of pattern can have a negative effect on your biological clock.

In order to get a good night's sleep, here are some things you can do:

- Set a regular sleep schedule.
- Do not exercise before bedtime.
- Avoid caffeine, nicotine, alcohol, and large meals before bedtime.
- Do not take naps after 3 P.M.
- Create a sleeping environment.
- Establish a relaxation ritual, such as taking a bath before bedtime.

Sometimes, though, you cannot sleep because you have to work the night shift. If possible, try to avoid that, but if you must, here are some steps to make it easier on your body:

- Increase the total time you sleep by sleeping more and adding naps.
- Use bright lights in your workplace.
- Reduce the sound and light distractions during your daytime sleep.
- Drink caffeine only during the first part of your shift.

Getting sleep is essential to having a healthy heart.

5. NURTURE HEALTHY RELATIONSHIPS

I was having a particularly difficult time with Roberto. Then, out of nowhere, I felt an unusual pain in my shoulder that radiated to my chest. It scared me because my mother had had a heart attack and I thought that perhaps this was how it felt. I did not know what to do. I calmed myself down and realized that I was just having a muscle spasm from the tension that I was feeling. —Nancy

BEING ALONE (THAT IS, SOCIAL ISOLATION) IS ASSOCIATED WITH blood pressure problems in men and women. Additionally, in men, it causes a higher cholesterol response, which may put them at risk of heart attack and other heart-related illnesses. Other research has shown that women who are married and in good relationships have fewer cardiovascular risk factors than other women.

Depression and stress are two of the consequences of unhealthy relationships, and both of these are major triggers for every type of heart problem. We know that the hormone oxytocin, the cuddling hormone, has an important effect on women and their well-being. We also know that men who rank high on measures of hostility and internal anger are more likely to have coronary heart disease.

Healthy relationships require work. No relationship is characterized by unending bliss, so when the usual conflicts crop up, we must resolve them in a positive way. *Aguantando* (accepting a situation out of a sense of responsibility) can be carried to an extreme that is damaging to all involved. Healthy relationships reflect mutual affection and respect. Those are the factors that keep a heart healthy.

6. HAVE A REGULAR SOURCE OF HEALTH CARE

When the surgeon came out of the operating room, he smiled and said that the procedure had been successful. He added that Mom was so small that it might have been better to do the procedure in a children's hospital. —Mark

I have ended up in the emergency room so many times with this condition. By now the ambulance should just park outside my house. —Myrna

AT THIS MOMENT, WHEN HEALTH CARE IS CHANGING SO dramatically, you need to have a health care provider you can talk to—and one who will listen to you. A recent study found that, even when given a diagnosis that required follow-up, Hispanics were less likely to schedule a follow-up visit. What increased the likelihood of pursuing treatment and follow-up was finding a health care provider who understood the language and the culture. Take the time to find someone you trust.

If you do have problems with your heart, your health care provider will send you to a cardiologist. A cardiologist is a physician who went through six to eight years of additional medical training to understand how to take care of your heart. Your cardiologist will be the health care provider most up-to-date on the treatment options for you. Do not wait to find one.

The problem with waiting is that the longer you wait, the more invasive the procedure will be to protect your health. There is much that can be done in health care today, but you need to be engaged and proactive in order to benefit from the advances.

7. KEEP A HEALTH JOURNAL

ALTHOUGH ELECTRONIC MEDICAL RECORDS ARE A GROWING PART OF our health care system, you also need to keep track of your own health history. You can do this by using any system that you want—manual or electronic—but you need to do it. When you get sick or are in an emergency situation, that is definitely not the time to struggle to recall the details of your health history. And you *will be asked to* give your medical history and a complete list of all your medications including the doses you take.

You can use the tools in Part III of this book to organize and maintain your health information.

8. CHERISH YOUR SPIRITUAL LIFE

FAITH HAS A STRONG IMPACT ON THE HEART. AT CRITICAL TIMES IN life, people reach for their religious roots as a source of strength and solace. As Hispanics, our sense of faith—regardless of our particular faith or whether we are currently practicing that faith—sustains us.

Faith helps to heal and restore the heart.

9. TAKE YOUR MEDICATIONS

Sara could not afford all her medications. Since she took so many, she decided that she would just stop taking one of them. She narrowed her decision to whether to take the medicines for diabetes or the medicine to control her cholesterol. It was not an easy choice, but she decided to take the medicine to control her cholesterol since she did not want to have a heart attack.

IN THE AREA OF HEART DISEASE, THE ADVANCES IN MEDICINES OVER the last twenty years have dramatically changed how we treat conditions of the heart. Today coronary artery bypass grafting (CABG) and heart transplants are much less frequent than they were years ago.

In our community, I sometimes hear people say that they do not want to take their medications because they are not natural. My response is that natural is not necessarily healthy. Arsenic is natural, but it can accumulate in your body and kill you. Others tell me they feel safer taking medications that they can buy in another country or over the counter. The reality is that if a medicine is not sold in the United States, you should not take it because it has not met the strict safety standards that have been established to protect you. Medicines—both prescription and over-the-counter (OTC)—help our bodies do their work. If you are prescribed particular medications, you need to take them. If you think you are having a bad reaction to a medicine, then you must let your health care provider know about that reaction so you can be advised as to what you should do.

Depending on your health and other medications that you are taking, it may be good for you to talk to your health care provider about whether you should be taking a low-dose aspirin once a day. The U.S. Preventive Services Task Force (USPSTF) recommends that men 45 to 79 years old and women 55 to 79 years old talk to their health care providers about whether the benefits of taking aspirin outweigh the potential harm. Research to date confirms that taking low-dose aspirin lowers the risk of heart attack in men, while it lowers the risk of stroke in women.

10. LISTEN TO YOUR BODY

Jaime knew that there was something wrong. He looked at himself in the mirror and saw a man of average weight, who ran regularly, and ate a healthy diet. However, he was unable to exercise as he usually did and just did not feel well. He called his internist, who referred him to a cardiologist for a preliminary test. The results of the test were fine, and his internist told Jaime that he had nothing to worry about. He told the internist that he still did not feel right and he was especially worried because his father had died of a heart attack at an early age. His internist told him, "Stop worrying. It's all in your head." Jaime decided he needed a primary care doctor who would listen to him and not just dismiss what he was saying. He found a new internist, who referred him to another cardiologist. The new cardiologist explained that because the results of the preliminary test were good, Jaime would have to pay for the additional tests in cash, because the insurance company would not cover the cost. The cardiologist also pointed out that there was a relatively small chance that the new tests would uncover a problem. Jaime then asked the new cardiologist, "What would you do if you were me?" and the doctor said, "You know your body better than anyone else. If you're worried, take the extra test. At the very least, the added expense will buy you some peace of mind." When the results came back, Jaime's cardiologist told him that he needed to have bypass surgery right away because he was on the verge of having a heart attack.

BE AWARE OF CHANGES IN YOUR BODY AND WHAT MIGHT HAVE caused them. No one knows you as well you can and should know yourself. So, to stay healthy, be aware of how you feel. When your body talks to you, listen and act.

To recap, here is the 10-Point Program for Health. Follow this and you will be doing your best to keep your heart healthy.

10-POINT PROGRAM FOR HEALTH

1. Stay away from smoke and toxic air.
2. Keep moving.
3. Eat and drink for a healthy heart.
4. Get enough sleep.
5. Nurture healthy relationships.
6. Have a regular source of health care.
7. Keep a health journal.
8. Cherish your spiritual life.
9. Take your medications.
10. Listen to your body.

Part Two

JUST THE FACTS

WHEN WE SAY *HEART PROBLEMS* OR *HEART DISEASE*, THESE TERMS encompass many different kinds of diagnoses. Part II has two sections. In the first section are the facts about the most frequently asked about conditions. The second section gives you an understanding of the different tests that are used for diagnosis and some of the procedures that are used to treat heart conditions.

～You say I have…

Aneurysm

ALSO KNOWN AS
abdominal aortic aneurysm, or AAA, aortic aneurysm, berry aneurysm, brain aneurysm, cerebral aneurysm, peripheral aneurysm, and thoracic aortic aneurysm, or TAA

Q *Que pasa?*
This refers to a bulge in an artery. It is most common in the wall of the aorta. The area where there is a bulge will become weak and, over time, the aneurysm will either burst or cause a tear in the artery wall. This can cause internal bleeding, a blood clot, or a stroke. The two major types of aortic aneurysms are abdominal aortic aneurysms (AAAs), which occur in the abdomen, and thoracic aortic aneurysms (TAAs), which occur in the chest. AAAs are 3 times more common than TAAs. Men are more likely to have an AAA than are women.

Other types of aneurysms are less common. These include cerebral, brain, or berry aneurysm, which are in the brain; and peripheral aneurysms, which may be located in the popliteal (back of the thighs and behind the knees), femoral (groin), or carotid (on either side of the neck) arteries.

CAUSES AND PREVENTION

There is no single cause for a person to develop an aneurysm. Some known factors that can cause the walls of an artery to weaken are smoking, uncontrolled high blood pressure, atherosclerosis, and injury (such as a car accident). People over the age of 65 are also more likely to have an aneurysm. Additionally, people who have vasculitis (inflammation of the blood vessels) are at risk for AAA, and people with certain genetic disorders are more likely to develop a TAA. If someone in your family has had an AAA, then your chances of having one before age 65 is greater than that of someone who has no family history of the disease.

Q *Do I have a problem?*
Most of the time, an AAA or a TAA develops slowly, and there are no symptoms until the aneurysm becomes large or ruptures. Aneurysms are usually discovered when a person has a CT scan for some other condition.

Q *What can I do?*
At a minimum, you should avoid smoking and tobacco smoke, make sure that your blood pressure is under control, and control your cholesterol. If an AAA is small (less than 2 inches [5 cm]), your health care provider will probably recommend that it be monitored to see if it gets bigger or begins to grow at a fast rate. If the AAA is larger than 2 inches (5 cm), you may be given medicines to make it easier for blood to flow through your arteries. In more advanced cases, your health care provider will refer you to a cardiothoracic surgeon (a physician who addresses the heart, lungs, chest, and aorta) or a vascular surgeon (a

physician who focuses on the aorta and the blood vessels, but not the heart or the brain). The most important step is to maintain regular visits and communication with your health care provider.

Angina

ALSO KNOWN AS
acute coronary syndrome, angina pectoris, chest pain, coronary artery spasms, microvascular angina, Prinzmetal's angina, stable or common angina, unstable angina, and variant angina

------

*Q**Que pasa?***
Angina is the name given to pain that you feel in your chest. It is your body's way of letting you know that the muscles of your heart are not getting enough oxygen-rich blood. It is a warning sign, not a disease. Sometimes people think they have gas or indigestion when it is really angina. All this emphasizes the importance of knowing your body.

There are different kinds of angina. *Stable angina* has a regular pattern and lasts for a few minutes (5 minutes or less) and goes away. After a while, you learn what you have to do to make it go away, as the episodes are similar. Usually you need some combination of rest and medication. Angina is typically brought on by overexerting yourself, emotional stress, exposure to very hot or cold temperatures, heavy meals, or smoking. *Unstable angina* is when you experience pain without exertion and you do not feel better by either resting or taking medicine. The pain is unexpected and can last as long as 30 minutes. It requires immediate treatment in an emergency room, as it may be a warning sign of a heart attack. *Variant (Prinzmetal's) angina* is rare and occurs when you are at rest, usually between midnight and the early morning. It is usually treated with medication. *Microvascular angina* is more severe, and medicines may not make it feel better. It also lasts for a longer time period and may indicate that you have coronary microvascular disease (MVD). It is first noticed during routine daily activities and times of mental or emotional stress.

CAUSES AND PREVENTION
Angina may be a symptom of coronary heart disease, coronary artery disease, or coronary microvascular disease (MVD). It occurs in roughly the same proportion of men and women.

Q Do I have a problem?
If you have chest pains, you should be checked by your health care provider. Chest pains can be caused by many things: for example, a muscle that you pulled, a panic attack, a blockage in an artery in the lung (a pulmonary embolism), a lung infection, or even indigestion.

Q What can I do?
It is best to see your health care provider to find out what is causing the pain and what to do to reduce the pain. The most important thing to remember is not to ignore the pain; pain is how your body lets you know that something is not right.

Arrhythmia

ALSO KNOWN AS
dysrhythmia

_Q_ *Que pasa?*
This is when your heart does not have a steady rhythm.
When you have an arrhythmia, the heart may have extra
beats or beat too fast (tachycardia), in an unpredictable manner,
or too slow (bradycardia). This usually means that the electrical
signals in your heart are not traveling in a systematic or pre-
dictable manner.

The major arrhythmias from fast heartbeats are called *supraven-*
tricular arrhythmias. These include atrial fibrillation (fast and irregular beats), atrial flutter (fast and regular beats), and paroxysmal
supraventicular tachycardia (PSVT—very fast beats that begin
and end suddenly). PSVT includes Wolff-Parkinson-White syndrome, in which the rapid heartbeats result from an extra electrical pathway.

Unpredictable beats due to problems in the lower heart chambers are called *ventricular arrhythmias* and include ventricular
tachycardia and ventricular fibrillation (v-fib). These are very
serious and need to be looked at by a health care provider as soon
as possible.

CAUSES AND PREVENTION
Arrhythmias occur when there is a disruption in the functioning
of the cells that produce electrical signals in your heart.
Arrhythmias may occur because of exposure to toxic chemicals
(tobacco smoke or ozone), drinking too much alcohol, use of certain substances (caffeine, cocaine, amphetamines), stress or anger

(which causes the release of hormones and may raise blood pressure), an underlying health problem (previous heart attack, uncontrolled high blood pressure, underactive or overactive thyroid problem), or even problems of the heart that a person was born with (congenital).

Many people have arrhythmias, and about 2.2 million people have atrial fibrillation (see page 56). Most of the arrhythmias that are serious occur in people over 60 years old, while young people are more likely to have the rarer types, such as PSVT or Wolff-Parkinson-White syndrome.

Q *Do I have a problem?*

It depends on how severe the problem is. In most cases the problem is mild and a person does not need treatment, while in other cases the disruption in the flow of blood can damage the body.

Atherosclerosis

ALSO KNOWN AS
arteriosclerotic vascular disease, or ASVD.
See coronary artery disease on page 64.

Q *Que pasa?*

If you have this common health problem, your arteries become clogged or blocked with fat, cholesterol, calcium, and other substances found in the blood. The combination of these substances is called *plaque,* and over time plaque accumulates on the walls of the arteries. There are many reasons why plaque builds up there, but most of the research suggests that little nicks in the arteries act as hooks and catch the plaque as it travels through the artery. Over time, the amount of plaque increases and hardens, creating a blockage. When there is a blockage, it is hard for your arteries to carry the oxygen-rich blood to the different parts of your body. The location of the blockage is used to give the condition a more specific name. For example, when the blood is blocked in the arteries that go to your legs, arms, and pelvis, it is called peripheral arterial disease (PAD). When plaque builds up in the arteries on each side of your neck, it is called carotid artery disease. These arteries bring blood to your brain, and when they become blocked it can lead to a stroke. You do not get atherosclerosis all at once. It is a disease that often begins when you are a child and continues to develop throughout your life. The older you are, the faster it develops.

CAUSES AND PREVENTION

We do not know what causes atherosclerosis. There are many theories about this, but none that establishes the definitive cause. Scientists are trying to find out how arteries become damaged, how plaque develops and changes over time, and what happens when a section of plaque breaks open.

Even though we do not have all the answers, there are certain factors that increase the chances that you will develop atherosclerosis. Some of these we cannot change: for example, if members of our family had heart disease, getting older, and the like. At the same time, there are other parts of our life we can change to make ourselves less prone to atherosclerosis. Those are the ones that we already know: Do not smoke, increase physical activity, eat healthy foods, and eat in moderation. Additionally, if you have hypertension or diabetes, it is very important to keep these conditions under control. And while we may make the excuse that some of our habits are rooted in our culture or that everything is in our genes, neither of those statements is an absolute. There is much that we can do now in our lives so we can enjoy a healthy future. That means we have to change some of the things we are doing now.

Q *Do I have a problem?*

For some people, the first sign that they have atherosclerosis is that they have a heart attack or stroke. Other people may feel numbness or pain because a part of their body is not getting enough blood. Sometimes, dangerous infections may occur because people do not realize that they have a problem.

Q *What can I do?*

If you are concerned about your risk, you should see your health care provider and discuss what can be done to make you better. Treatment typically requires you to change some of the things in your life (stop smoking, start or increase the intensity or duration of your exercise program, eat healthy, etc.) and take the medications prescribed by your health care provider. Sometimes you may have to undergo some procedures to help your body get better. Taking care of yourself and seeing your health care provider on a regular basis can reduce the likelihood that you will have complications from atherosclerosis.

Atrial fibrillation

ALSO KNOWN AS
AF, a-fib, or auricular fibrillation

> I will do whatever I must to get better. When my
> condition gets bad, my heart beats over 200 times a
> minute. It is unbelievable. My heart beats so forcefully
> that you can see how it makes my blouse move up
> and down. It is scary to see and scary to feel. —Yvette

Q ***Que pasa?***
The heart beats in a fast and irregular way. This makes the upper part of the heart (the atria) quiver very fast (fibrillate) and does not allow for the normal pumping of blood into the lower chambers (the ventricles). As a result, the blood accumulates in the upper chambers and the synchronized movement of the upper and lower parts of the heart get out of sync.

There are 3 types of atrial fibrillation. When the abnormal electrical signals and rapid heart rate begin suddenly and then stop on their own, it is called *paroxysmal atrial fibrillation*. If the abnormal heart rhythm can be stopped with treatment, it is called *persistent atrial fibrillation*. When the usual treatments cannot restore a normal heart rhythm, a person has *permanent atrial fibrillation*.

CAUSES AND PREVENTION

Sometimes AF occurs for no apparent reason. In the majority of cases, someone who has AF also has at least one other related condition, such as high blood pressure, coronary artery disease, heart failure, rheumatic heart disease, mitral valve disorder, overactive thyroid gland, or heavy alcohol use. AF is also more common in older adults.

When you have AF, it means that the electrical system in your heart is not functioning as it should be. The electrical signals seem to travel in unpredictable ways and the heart begins to beat very fast (100 to 175 times a minute in the adult heart). As a result, the amount of blood that goes to the organs and tissues is disrupted; sometimes they may get too little blood; at other times too much.

Q *Do I have a problem?*

AF can occur once or it can be an ongoing problem. Your health care provider will most likely refer you to a cardiologist who will help you manage or eliminate the condition. Medications, medical procedures, and changes in how you live your life may all be part of your treatment plan.

Cardiomyopathy

Q *Que pasa?*

This is when the heart muscle has a disease. The 4 major types of heart-muscle disease are dilated cardiomyopathy, hypertrophic cardiomyopathy, restrictive cardiomyopathy, and arrhythmogenic right ventricular dysplasia (ARVD). Each of these types also has other names that are more descriptive. For example, other names for dilated cardiomyopathy includes alcoholic, congestive, familial, idiopathic, ischemic, peripartum, or primary cardiomyopathy. Hypertrophic cardiomyopathy may also be called asymmetric septal, familial hypertrophic, hypertrophic nonobstructive, hypertrophic obstructive, or idiopathic hypertrophic cardiomyopathy. Regardless of the type, as the condition gets worse, the heart is less able to pump blood or beat in a regular way. Without adequate blood, the person may experience either heart failure or arrhythmia.

You can either inherit this condition or get it as a result of infection, presence of another disease (high blood pressure), excessive use of alcohol, or exposure to a toxin (such as cobalt).

CAUSES AND PREVENTION

For most people, the cause of the condition is unknown, although there is some information about each type. Specifically, *dilated cardiomyopathy* is usually found in men ages 20 to 60. It is more common among African Americans than among non-Hispanic whites. In this condition, the heart muscle gets thin and starts to stretch. Left untreated, it can lead to heart valve problems, arrhythmias, and blood clots in the heart. For half the cases, there is no known cause, and for nearly a third the condition is inherited. The remaining cases are due to a variety of reasons, including coronary artery disease, heart attack, diabetes, thyroid disease, viral hepatitis, HIV, infections (especially viral infections that inflame the heart muscle), alcohol, complications during the last month of pregnancy or within 5 months of giving birth, exposure to certain toxins (such as cobalt), certain drugs (such as cocaine and amphetamines), and two medicines used to treat cancer (doxorubicin and daunorubicin).

Hypertrophic cardiomyopathy occurs when the wall of the lower chamber (ventricle) thickens and in some instances stiffens. This condition is found in 1 in 500 people and occurs just as frequently in men and as in women. It is also the most likely cause of sudden cardiac arrest (SCA) in young people. The condition is usually inherited, although it can develop in older people or in people with uncontrolled high blood pressure.

Restrictive cardiomyopathy is diagnosed when the normal tissue that makes up the heart muscle is replaced with scar tissue or other abnormal tissue. This is more common among older adults and may be caused by a variety of conditions, such as excessive iron accumulation in the body, abnormal buildup of protein in the body, and connective tissue disorders.

Arrhythmogenic right ventricular dysplasia (ARVD) is a rare condition in which the muscle in the lower-right chamber dies and is replaced by scar tissue. This typically is seen in teens or young adults. It is believed to be inherited.

Q *Do I have a problem?*

It is hard to tell, as some people have no symptoms and do not require treatment. Knowing if you are at risk is important to maintaining your health. The risk factors include the following:

- A family history of heart problems, including cardio-myopathy, heart failure, or sudden cardiac arrest (SCA).
- A disease or condition that can lead to cardiomyopa-thy, such as coronary artery disease, heart attack, or a viral infection that inflames the heart muscle.
- Diabetes, other metabolic diseases, or severe excess weight.
- Diseases that can damage the heart.
- Alcoholism.
- Uncontrolled high blood pressure.

In some cases, cardiomyopathy that goes untreated will progress to heart failure. Be alert to the signs of heart failure (see page 63) and see your health care provider if you feel that cardiomyopathy is a concern.

Q *What can I do?*

Your next steps will be taken under the guidance of your cardiologist and will include treating any underlying conditions. Additionally, you need to follow the basics, that is, stop smoking and avoid exposure to smoke (secondhand and thirdhand), improve what and how you eat, limit your use of alcohol, do not use illegal substances, identify the level of physical activity that will be most beneficial, and nurture healthy relationships. People with hypertrophic cardiomyopathy will be given very specific information on the types and amounts of physical activity that they can engage in. These steps, combined with taking your medications, will be sufficient to control the condition for most people. In some cases, your cardiologist may want to implant a pacemaker (to improve your heart rhythm) or an implantable cardioverter defibrillator (ICD). In more severe cases, open-heart surgery may offer the best solution.

Congenital heart defects

ALSO KNOWN AS
congenital heart disease, heart defects, and
congenital cardiovascular malformations

Q *Que pasa?*
When a heart does not develop properly before birth, the person is born with a congenital heart defect. This occurs in 8 out of every 1,000 newborns, or about 35,000 newborns annually. Today about 1 million adults in the United States have a congenital heart defect.

CAUSES AND PREVENTION

In the majority of cases, the cause of congenital heart defects is not known. All that is known is that for some reason the heart developed in a way that was not expected. There are instances where we can see a stronger causal connection with respect to the congenital heart defect. For example, half of the babies with Down syndrome have a congenital heart defect. Additionally, women who smoke during pregnancy are more likely to have a baby with a congenital heart defect.

Q *Do I have a problem?*
Severe defects are identified during pregnancy or soon after birth. You probably do not have a congenital heart defect if you have reached adulthood and have never been told that you have a congenital heart defect. Keep in mind that, in many instances, it is difficult for a health care provider to pick up whether you have a congenital heart defect during a general physical exam. The exception is those cases where the defect

worsens, and as the heart has to work harder you develop symptoms that signal the need for further testing.

Congestive heart failure

ALSO KNOWN AS
CHF and heart failure

> When the doctor told me my mother had heart failure, I could feel my own heart sink. I didn't know what to say or think. All I could think was that there were only a few days left. I could not believe it. She had been fine just a few days before. —Carla

Que pasa?

First of all, this does not mean that your heart has failed; it does mean that your heart is not able to supply your body with the required blood flow. Specifically, heart failure is when your heart is unable to either fill up with blood or pump blood—or sometimes both—and, because of that, the other organs in your body cannot get enough blood to function properly.

Usually this does not happen all at once. Congestive heart failure (CHF) is a condition that gets worse over time. It can involve either or both sides of the heart. There are 5.7 million people in the United State with heart failure. Each year about 300,000 adults and children die from the condition. It is more common in people over 65 and is the most frequently mentioned reason for hospital visits among people enrolled in Medicare. It is also more common among African Americans, people who are overweight, and men.

CAUSES AND PREVENTION

In most cases CHF is the result of other conditions that are known to damage the heart, such as coronary heart disease (CHD), high blood pressure, diabetes, cardiomyopathy, problems with the heart valve, irregular heartbeats (arrythmias), congenital heart defects, certain treatments for cancer (such as radiation and chemotherapy), thyroid disorders (having either too much or too little thyroid hormone in the body), alcohol abuse, cocaine and other illegal drug use, HIV/AIDS, too much vitamin E, and obstructive sleep apnea.

Q *Do I have a problem?*

Since there is no cure for heart failure, the earlier that it is diagnosed and treated, the better the outcome. You should know the signs of heart failure. They include:

- Shortness of breath or trouble breathing.
- Fatigue (tiredness).
- Swelling in the feet, ankles, legs, and abdomen.

In rare instances, there may be swelling in the veins of your neck. As the fluid builds up in the body, the heart gets weaker and the symptoms get worse. Other signs and symptoms as the heart failure worsens may include dizziness, light-headedness, fainting during physical activity, chest pain, arrhythmias, and heart murmur (an extra or unusual sound heard during a heartbeat).

It is hard for your health care provider to know if you are in the early stages of congestive heart failure since there is no single test to diagnose the condition. To gather information, your health care provider will listen to your heart for sounds that are not normal, listen to your lungs to make sure that they are clear, and look for swelling. If your health care provider is concerned, you will be referred to a cardiologist for further assessment.

Q *What can I do?*
Whether or not you have been diagnosed with CHF, the key steps you should take include making a renewed commitment to living a healthier life; avoiding all toxic substances, such as tobacco and illegal drugs; not drinking alcohol; maintaining a healthy weight; and staying physically active on a regular basis. If you are diagnosed with CHF, the goal is to do everything you can to prevent your heart failure from getting worse. Besides the key health steps, you will have to monitor the type and the amount of liquids you drink, take your medications as directed, and get ongoing care. This will make it possible for you to live longer and enjoy your life.

Coronary artery disease

ALSO KNOWN AS
CAD, coronary heart disease, atherosclerosis, hardening of the arteries, heart disease, ischemic heart disease, and narrowing of the arteries

---

Q *Que pasa?*
When the body recognizes that there is an injury or infection, it sets into motion an inflammation response. This response works to protect you and quickly heal whatever is damaged. When the walls of an artery become damaged, the inflammation response gets activated. For some unknown reason, this also helps plaque to grow. CAD occurs when some part or parts

of your arteries are partially or fully blocked, due to the accumulation of plaque (a combination of fat, cholesterol, calcium, and other substances found in the blood). This blockage also makes it more likely that blood clots will form in your arteries. Blood clots also can partially or completely block blood flow.

When blood flow to your heart muscle is reduced or blocked, it can lead to angina, heart failure, and even a heart attack. This is the major cause of death for everyone—both men and women—in the United States. When plaque forms in the smallest arteries of the heart, it is called coronary microvascular disease (MVD). Each year about 500,000 men and women in the United States die from CAD.

CAUSES AND PREVENTION

Smoking, high blood pressure, unhealthy blood cholesterol levels, uncontrolled diabetes, insufficient amounts of physical activity, and metabolic syndrome are only some of the factors that can damage the inside of your arteries. The damage causes little nicks where plaque can accumulate as the body tries to heal the injured area. The risk of developing CAD increases for men over 45 and women over 55. The health of family members may give you a clue as to your risk, too. If you have any male family members who were diagnosed with CAD before age 55 or female family members who were diagnosed with CAD before age 65, you are at increased risk for CAD.

There is much you can do to reduce your risk and, in many cases, decrease the likelihood of triggering genetic tendencies to develop CAD. These include avoiding toxic substances (smoke, high levels of ozone, alcohol, etc.), controlling your blood pressure, increasing and maintaining physical activity, eating in a healthy way, taking your medications as directed, seeing your health care provider on a regular basis, focusing on healthy relationships, reducing stress, and treating sleep apnea.

Q Do I have a problem?

In some cases, there are no signs or symptoms of CAD. The common symptoms (pain in your chest, shortness of breath, etc.) may be relatively mild until the plaque builds up and there is more blockage. As the level of blockage increases, you are more likely to experience heart failure, heart attack, and/or irregular heartbeats (arrhythmias).

Given your health history and risk factors, your health care provider may do some ongoing monitoring of your heart. This usually includes listening to your heart and lungs, doing an electrocardiogram (EKG), determining your level of cholesterol and triglycerides through a blood test, and taking your blood pressure. Some health care providers may want to do a blood test to determine your level of C-reactive protein (CRP). When CRP levels are high, it means that the inflammation response has kicked in. Although that is useful information, increased CRP levels can also be due to injury or infection in some other part of your body. Scientists are starting to further investigate the relationship between CRP and CAD.

Q What can I do?

Be proactive and know what your risk factors are. Additionally, when your health care provider prescribes medications, ask what they are for so that you understand how they will help you. Some medications are to treat another condition that, if not controlled, may damage your heart, such as hypertension and diabetes; others may help prevent or delay the onset of CAD by helping to keep your arteries healthy and clear.

Coronary microvascular disease

ALSO KNOWN AS
MVD, cardiac syndrome X, and nonobstructive coronary heart disease

---

Q *Que pasa?*
The problem in coronary microvascular disease is that in the smallest coronary arteries that surround the heart, there is an increase in plaque. Surprisingly, this increase in plaque does not create blockages. This condition is more common in women. Research into this condition is relatively new. We do know that men and women who have diabetes or high blood pressure often have MVD. Additionally, younger women with hypertension or lower-than-normal levels of estrogen *before* menopause are more likely to develop MVD. This may be due to factors that reduce normal levels of estrogen, such as mental or emotional stress or problems with the normal functioning of the ovaries.

CAUSES AND PREVENTION

There is very little known about MVD. In 2006 the National Heart, Lung, and Blood Institute reported some of the first findings from the WISE Study (Women's Ischemia Syndrome Evaluation). Specifically, the institute's report stated:

> In as many as 3 million U.S. women with coronary heart disease, cholesterol plaque may not build up into major blockages, but instead spreads evenly throughout the artery wall. As a result, diagnostic coronary angiogra-

phy reveals that these women have "clear" arteries—
no blockages—incorrectly indicating low risk.

There have been no studies on how to prevent MVD. Taking the steps to lead a healthier life should reduce your risk of developing this condition. MVD is hard to diagnose because the tests and procedures used to diagnose coronary heart disease usually focus on blockages in large arteries and are not sensitive enough to pick up MVD.

Q *What can I do?*
Since it is not known if prevention of MVD is different from preventing coronary heart disease (CHD), you should focus on doing all you can to stay as healthy as you can. You need to take control of your health and take all the steps that will increase your health—avoid toxic substances (smoke, ozone, excessive alcohol, etc.), eat healthy food, do more exercise, reduce stress, take your medications for high blood pressure and diabetes, and the like. If you have anemia, it is important to treat it, because anemia has a negative impact on the cells that are responsible for repairing damaged blood vessels. Most important is to know yourself so that you know when to seek medical help.

Endocarditis

ALSO KNOWN AS
infective endocarditis, or IE

Q *Que pasa?*
This is an infection in the inner lining of your heart chambers and valves. It occurs when bacteria, fungi, or other

microbes enter the body and travel through the bloodstream to your heart. Once the microbes settle in your heart, they can cause damage. Endocarditis can develop quickly (acute infective endocarditis) or slowly (subacute infective endocarditis). As the condition progresses, the bacteria that have multiplied in your heart grow and start to form clumps. These clumps, called *vegetations*, are dangerous because they are likely to break off and travel to the lungs (causing a pulmonary embolism), the kidneys, the spleen, and other parts of the body. When they travel to the brain, these clumps are called *emboli*, and they can cause seizures, strokes, localized infections (brain abscesses), or widespread infections (meningitis).

CAUSES AND PREVENTION

Most of the people who develop endocarditis have a heart that has been compromised by damage, artificial heart valves, congenital heart defects, and/or medical devices that have been implanted in their heart or blood vessels. IE develops in people who engage in activities that allow for microbes to enter their bloodstream, such as having unhealthy teeth and gums, injecting intravenous drugs, piercing the body, or using catheters or medical devices for longer periods than what is recommended. If you think you are at risk for IE, be sure to tell your dentist. Some of those at risk may be asked to take antibiotics before undergoing most dental procedures.

Q *Do I have a problem?*
It is hard to tell whether or not you have a problem, because the key symptoms of fever or tiredness that does not go away are found in many other common conditions. Additionally, since the condition may have different causes, the

symptoms may vary from one person to another, and even for the same person from one episode to another. Some of the other symptoms include:

1. Shortness of breath or a lingering cough.
2. A new heart murmur or a change in an existing one.
3. Changes in your skin: for example, overall paleness; small, painful, red or purplish bumps under the skin on the fingers or toes; small, dark, painless, flat spots on the palms of the hands or the soles of the feet; tiny spots under the fingernails, on the whites of the eyes, on the roof of the mouth, and inside the cheeks, or on the chest.
3. Nausea (feeling sick to your stomach), vomiting, a decrease in appetite, a sense of fullness with discomfort on the upper left side of the abdomen, or weight loss with or without a change in appetite.
4. Blood in the urine.
5. Swelling in the feet, legs, or abdomen.

Since there is no single test or symptom of endocarditis, your health care provider will have to conduct a series of tests to determine what is causing your symptoms. If endocarditis is suspected, your blood tests will be a key source of information. Over a 24-hour period, you will be asked to provide several blood samples. The bacteria in those samples will be allowed to grow to determine which medication will be most effective in treating your condition. Although there are cases of IE in which, based on blood tests, it seems that no bacteria are present (called culture-negative endocarditis), the person will still be given antibiotics.

Q *What can I do?*
In some cases you will need to take antibiotics for several weeks. Some people with IE have to undergo a procedure to repair damage to the heart valves.

Heart attack

ALSO KNOWN AS
myocardial infarction, or MI, acute myocardial infarction, or AMI, acute coronary syndrome, coronary thrombosis, and coronary occlusion

> Guillermo never had anything good to say about Dr. Sanchez. He would tell anyone who would listen to him that Dr. Sanchez was a terrible physician. After all, he had gone to see him, had a full physical, been told that all his tests were negative, and then 48 hours later he found himself in the emergency room having a heart attack. He blamed Dr. Sanchez for not diagnosing his heart problems.

Q *Que pasa?*
The blood flow to your heart is blocked and the heart muscle does not get the blood it needs to function. The muscle will begin to die if steps are not taken to get the blood flowing to the area.

CAUSES AND PREVENTION
Most heart attacks are due to coronary artery disease (CAD). The risk for a heart attack is greater among men over 45 and women over 55 or after menopause. Additionally, your risk increases if your father or a brother was diagnosed with CAD before 55 years

of age or if your mother or a sister was diagnosed with CAD before 65 years of age. While you cannot control these factors, you can control other risk factors. Specifically, you should quit smoking *and* stay away from smoke (secondhand and thirdhand), control your high blood pressure, reduce excess weight, increase physical activity, and manage your diabetes. Once you have had a heart attack, you need to follow the life plan and treatment that you develop with your health care provider to care for your heart.

Q Do I have a problem?

Hollywood has done us all a disservice by having us believe that people having a heart attack clutch their chest and fall over. In fact, the symptoms of heart attack vary from person to person. Men and women also tend to have different clusters of symptoms. And even when you have survived one heart attack, the symptoms may be different if you have another one.

Usually there is pain or discomfort in the middle of the chest that lasts for more than a few minutes. The feeling may be of pressure, squeezing, pain, or fullness. Sometimes the signs of a heart attack are mistaken for indigestion or heartburn. Other common symptoms include:

1. Upper body discomfort in one or both arms, the back, the neck, the jaw, or the stomach.
2. Shortness of breath, which often occurs with or before chest discomfort.
3. Nausea (you feel like throwing up), vomiting, lightheadedness, or fainting.
4. Breaking out in a cold sweat.

Women are more than twice as likely as men to experience nausea, vomiting, or indigestion.

Q *What can I do?*
Get emergency help as soon as possible. If you think you or someone you are with is having a heart attack, call 9-1-1 so that emergency personnel can stabilize you. The longer you wait to get help, the more damage there will be to your heart. Do not drive yourself anywhere.

Heart murmur

Q *Que pasa?*
Your heart is making an unusual sound that is like a rasping or whooshing sound. Most of the time a sound that is different is okay—that is, innocent or harmless. These may be called normal, benign, functional, physiologic, Still's, or flow murmurs. They are not a cause for concern. A heart murmur that may be a problem is an abnormal or pathologic heart murmur.

The sound of the typical heartbeat is "lub-DUPP" or "lub-DUB." This is the sound of the opening and closing of the valves in your heart as your blood flows through. It is also the sound that your health care provider hears with a stethoscope. The "lub" sound is when the lower part of your heart pumps the blood out of the heart and the "DUB" or "DUPP" sound is when the heart fills with blood.

CAUSES AND PREVENTION

Adults who have heart murmurs are likely to have had their heart valves damaged due to infection or disease (such as rheumatic fever, endocarditis, calcification, or mitral valve prolapse). Sometimes, as we get older, the heart valves get hard and do not work as well. Problems can occur because a valve does not close tightly (mitral regurgitation) or the timing is off when the valves close (split S2).

Q Do I have a problem?

Since most heart murmurs are harmless, most people have no signs or symptoms. Some harmless murmurs are due to conditions that must be treated, such as anemia, fever, or hyperthyroidism. If the heart murmur is abnormal, some possible symptoms include the following:

1. A blue tinge on the skin, especially on the fingertips and inside the mouth
2. Shortness of breath
3. Excessive sweating
4. Chest pain
5. Dizziness or fainting
6. Feeling very tired

Your health care provider will listen to the sounds your heart makes and, depending on when the sound is heard, will classify the heart murmur as systolic (pumping blood out), diastolic (filling up with blood), or continuous (throughout the entire heartbeat). The sounds will also be classified by how loud they are. This is usually done using a 6-point scale with grade 1 indicating that it can barely be heard. This would be called a grade 1/VI murmur.

Q What can I do?

In most cases, treatment will not be necessary, as the heart murmur is harmless. In cases when there are concerns, you need to follow the treatment prescribed by your health care provider, which may consist of medications or a surgical procedure.

Heart palpitations

Q Que pasa?
This is when you feel that your heart is beating in a way that is different than usual. It could be that it feels like your heart is beating too fast or skipping a beat. You may feel this in your chest, throat, or neck. Palpitations are very common and, in most instances, they are not a cause for concern.

CAUSES AND PREVENTION
You can have palpitations for many reasons that are not related to heart problems, such as having very strong feelings of anxiety, fear, or panic; experiencing stress; engaging in strenuous physical activity; taking certain medications that have stimulants, like diet pills (amphetamines) and some decongestants; going through hormonal changes; consuming caffeine, alcohol, nicotine, or illegal drugs; and having certain medical conditions, such as thyroid disease, fever, dehydration, low blood sugar, or anemia. If you have heart disease (heart failure, valve problems, etc.), palpitations are likely to be related to an arrhythmia.

Q Do I have a problem?
You should discuss what you feel is a palpitation with your health care provider, especially if you feel dizzy or confused; get so light-headed that you think you may faint, or do faint; have trouble breathing or feel short of breath; have pain, pressure, or tightness in your chest, jaw, or arm; or are sweating more than usual.

Q *What can I do?*
You have to avoid whatever is triggering the palpitations. This may mean that you must avoid certain people in your life. Palpitations that are not due to a medical condition are a signal from your body that something is not good for you. The best thing to do is to listen to your body and avoid whatever is causing this reaction.

Heart valve disease

ALSO KNOWN AS
aortic regurgitation, aortic stenosis, aortic sclerosis, aortic valve disease, bicuspid aortic valve, congenital heart defect, congenital valve disease, mitral regurgitation, mitral stenosis, mitral valve disease, mitral valve prolapse, pulmonic regurgitation, pulmonic stenosis, pulmonic valve disease, tricuspid regurgitation, tricuspid stenosis, and tricuspid valve disease

---

Q *Que pasa?*
The many names for heart valve disease reflect that this disease occurs when at least 1 of 4 valves in your heart does not function because of 1 of 3 problems. The 4 valves in your heart are the tricuspid valve (between the right atrium and the right ventricle); the pulmonary valve (on the right side of the heart, between the right ventricle and the pulmonary artery; this carries blood to the lungs); the mitral valve (between the left atrium and the left ventricle); and the aortic valve (on the left side of the heart, between the left ventricle and the aorta; this carries blood to the body). Valve problems may be due to a backflow of blood when the valve cannot close tightly (regurgitation); thickening or stiffening so it cannot fully open (stenosis); or when

there is no opening for blood to pass through (atresia). Backflow problems usually occur when the flaps of the valve flop or bulge back into the upper heart chamber during a heartbeat. This is called *prolapse* and is most commonly a problem with the mitral valve. Some people are born with valve problems and others have a small problem that initially has no signs or symptoms, but worsens as they get older.

CAUSES AND PREVENTION

Many conditions may cause heart valve disease. These include injury to the heart (including heart attack), uncontrolled high blood pressure, heart failure, endocarditis, plaque buildup in the arteries, increased calcium deposits in men older than 65 and women over 75, rheumatic fever, infections, lupus and other autoimmune diseases, some medications, and radiation therapy in the chest. While you can steer clear of some of these factors, others you cannot avoid. A major risk factor for heart valve disease is being over 75 years old; 1 in 8 people over the age of 75 has at least moderate heart valve disease.

Q *Do I have a problem?*
You will need to see a cardiologist to know for certain whether you have a problem with the valves in your heart. An electrocardiogram (EKG) and chest x-ray will provide some basic information. An echocardiogram (echo) will provide vital information on the state of your valves and will be used to confirm the condition of your valves.

Q *What can I do?*
There are no medications to treat heart valve disease. You can and must protect the valves from further dam-

age and treat whatever other heart-related conditions you may have. If the valves are in very bad shape, then you will need a procedure to replace them.

High blood cholesterol

ALSO KNOWN AS
hypercholesterolemia and hyperlipidemia

Q Que pasa?
When you have too much cholesterol, you run a higher risk of developing heart disease. To function properly, your body needs cholesterol and a way to transport it throughout your body. Your body uses special cells to transport cholesterol. These cells have protein on the outside and fat (lipids) and cholesterol on the inside. These transporters are called lipoproteins. They are either low-density lipoproteins (LDLs) or high-density lipoproteins (HDLs). To have a desirable cholesterol level, you want your level of low-density lipoprotein (LDL) to be low and your level of high-density lipoprotein (HDL) to be high. Triglycerides are another substance in your blood that you need to know about. We are learning more about the relationship between the levels of cholesterol and having a healthy heart. Keep in mind that adults with desirable levels of cholesterol are also at risk of heart attacks. In fact, half of all heart attacks occur in people who have normal cholesterol levels. The role of triglycerides is also getting more attention.

CAUSES AND PREVENTION
It is not known what causes blood cholesterol levels to rise. In some families, high levels of cholesterol are due to an inherited

genetic condition (hypercholesterolemia). Generally speaking, men tend to have lower levels of HDL as compared to women. Additionally, women under 55 seem to have lower levels of LDL than men. Once women reach age 55, they tend to have the same levels of LDL as men.

To get healthier levels of cholesterol, you should eat foods without any trans fats (trans fatty acids) and fewer foods with saturated fat (meat, butter, cheese, etc.). It is also good not to smoke, to maintain a healthy weight, to engage in physical activity on a regular basis, and to control your high blood pressure and diabetes. In addition, if you want to have healthy levels of triglycerides you should avoid drinking too much alcohol and avoid eating foods high in carbohydrates.

Q *Do I have a problem?*

Most people do not have any signs or symptoms of high blood cholesterol. They learn they have a problem when they get back results from a blood test. To determine your HDL, LDL, total cholesterol level, and triglyceride level, you have to get a lipid (lipoprotein) profile or panel. For this blood test to be accurate, you cannot consume anything but water for 9 to 12 hours before taking the test. This means you cannot eat or drink anything but water until after you give a blood sample. If you cannot fast for that long, you can get a more limited test that will give you results of your total cholesterol and HDL. To make it even easier for you, there are home versions of both these tests that are FDA-approved. These home test kits are fast, accurate, and simple to use, and can give you results very quickly. Adults need to have their levels of cholesterol screened at least every five years and much more frequently if they have risk factors for heart disease. The chart that follows tells you what the numbers suggest.

Total Cholesterol Level	Total Cholesterol Category
Less than 200 mg/dL	Desirable
200–239 mg/dL	Borderline high
240 mg/dL and above	High

LDL Cholesterol Level	LDL Cholesterol Category
Less than 100 mg/dL	Optimal
100–129 mg/dL	Near optimal/above optimal
130–159 mg/dL	Borderline high
160–189 mg/dL	High
190 mg/dL and above	Very high

HDL Cholesterol Level	HDL Cholesterol Category
Less than 40 mg/dL disease	A major risk factor for heart
40–59 mg/dL	The higher, the better
60 mg/dL and above	Considered protective against heart disease

Triglycerides	Triglycerides Category
Less than 150 mg/dL	Desirable
150–199 mg/dL	Borderline high
200 mg/dL and above	High

What can I do?

Q While you cannot change some of the factors that increase your risk of developing unhealthy levels of cholesterol, such as your age or family history, you can follow the 10-Point Program for Health, spelled out in Part I.

High blood pressure

ALSO KNOWN AS
HBP or hypertension

) I can't believe I have high blood pressure. I am not
(overweight. I run. I play tennis. I am an active person.

—Consuelo

Q *Que pasa?*
This means that the pressure your heart has to exert against the walls of your bloods vessels is too high. One in 3 adults, or 72 million people in the United States, have high blood pressure. Blood pressure is stated using 2 numbers, such as 110 over 80, and written as 110/80 *mmHg* (mmHg stands for "millimeters of mercury"; this is how blood pressure is measured). The first number is the pressure when the heart beats (systolic pressure) and the second number is the pressure when the heart rests (diastolic pressure).

CAUSES AND PREVENTION
In most cases (95 percent), the cause of high blood pressure is unknown. This type of hypertension is called *essential, primary,* or *idiopathic hypertension.* For the remaining 5 percent of cases, the HBP is due to another condition and is called *secondary high blood pressure* or *secondary hypertension.* When only the first number (systolic) is high, the condition is called *isolated systolic hypertension* (ISH). ISH is as damaging as when both numbers are high and is common in older people. Nearly two-thirds of people over age 60 with high blood pressure have ISH. We also know that as people get older, blood pressure rises.

Some medications, such as birth control pills, hormone therapy, and asthma medicines, can raise blood pressure. Your blood pressure may also go up if you have chronic kidney disease, thyroid disease, or sleep apnea.

Q *Do I have a problem?*

You should be taking your blood pressure on a regular basis. You can do this at home, in many offices, in grocery stores, and, of course, wherever you go for health care. If your blood pressure is a concern, then you need to see your health care provider and develop a treatment plan. See the chart titled "Blood Pressure Levels in Adults" to determine whether you need to take steps to bring your blood pressure under control.

BLOOD PRESSURE LEVELS IN ADULTS (IN MMHG)

CATEGORY	SYSTOLIC (top or 1st number)		DIASTOLIC (bottom or 2nd number)
Low (hypotension)	Less than 90	or	Less than 60
Normal	Less than 120	and	Less than 80
Prehypertension	120–139	or	80–89
High blood pressure			
Stage 1	140–159	or	90–99
Stage 2	160 or higher	or	100 or higher

Q *What can I do?*

If you have high blood pressure, you need to take your medications as prescribed, monitor your blood pressure on a regular basis, and live your life in a way that supports good heart health.

Lung diseases

Que pasa?

Q Your heart and lung work together. When you have problems breathing, it affects how well your heart can do its work. That is why, when the air quality is bad, hospitals report that more people end up in the emergency room with heart problems. What you breathe in is what fills the oxygen-depleted cells that the heart pumps into the lungs. When you breathe in substances that are unhealthy, they fill your blood cells and are pumped by the heart throughout the body to all your organs and tissues. What goes in through your lungs goes straight to your heart and all your other organs.

For most of us, our lungs work well. Lungs make it possible to remove the carbon dioxide that cells produce and to bring in oxygen from the air. This essential gas exchange is the key function of the lungs. When your lungs work well, you can take in as much air as you need, you can blow out all the air in your lungs and do so as quickly as is necessary, you do not have any problems in removing carbon dioxide from cells or adding oxygen from the air to your blood, and your muscles are as strong as they need to be to be able to take each breath. When you cannot do one or more of these actions, it is very likely that you have lung disease.

CAUSES AND PREVENTION

There are dozens of lung diseases. These include asthma, chronic bronchitis, emphysema, COPD or chronic obstructive pulmonary disease, lung cancer, pneumonia, pulmonary embolism, and asbestos-related lung diseases. The majority of these result from exposure to toxic substances (tobacco, asbestos, ozone, drywall dust, etc.), allergens, bacteria and viruses, and radiation. A very small percentage of lung diseases are due to conditions that you are born with (congenital defect) or a genetic disorder.

Q *Do I have a problem?*
In order to know if you have a problem with your lungs, your health care provider will want to know your answers to the questions below.

1. Do you ever feel as if you cannot breathe in enough air? ☐ yes ☐ no
2. Does your chest feel tight sometimes? ☐ yes ☐ no
3. Are there times when you find yourself coughing or wheezing (a whistling sound when you breathe for no apparent reason)? ☐ yes ☐ no
4. Do you ever have chest pain? ☐ yes ☐ no
5. When you walk, do you get out of breath? ☐ yes ☐ no
6. Have you or has anyone in your family had asthma and/or allergies? ☐ yes ☐ no
7. Have you or has anyone in your family had heart disease? ☐ yes ☐ no
8. Have you or has anyone in your family ever smoked? ☐ yes ☐ no
9. Have you or has anyone in your family visited places where you may have been exposed to tuberculosis? ☐ yes ☐ no
10. Have you or has anyone in your family worked or lived in a place that exposed you to dust, fumes, or particles (like asbestos)? ☐ yes ☐ no

If you answered "yes" to some of these questions, your health care provider may want you to get some lung function tests. These tests are relatively simple and noninvasive. Once you have a diagnosis, you should take your medications as directed by your health care provider and take actions that will support your lung health.

Q ***What can I do?***
To avoid lung disease and to reduce the likelihood that lung disease will worsen, there are some key steps you can take. First, avoid exposure to toxic substances, such as tobacco smoke, ozone, dust, and radiation. In the case of smoke, this means that you should not smoke, be around people who are smoking, or inhale the leftover smells of smoke. It also means that while it may be a beautiful, sunny day outside, if the ozone level is code orange, red, or purple, you should seriously reconsider any outdoor plans.

Metabolic syndrome

ALSO KNOWN AS
dysmetabolic syndrome, hypertriglyceridemic waist, insulin resistance syndrome, obesity syndrome, and syndrome X

Q ***Que pasa?***
This is a cluster of risk factors that, when taken together, increase your risk of heart disease. It is a relatively new diagnosis for a condition that is found in almost 25 percent of the adults (47 million people) in the United States. Although it is found in the same proportions among in non-Hispanic white men and women, it is more common among African American women, Mexican American women, and South Asian men and women. Also at increased risk for metabolic syndrome are people who have diabetes, have a brother or sis-

ter or parent with diabetes, or women who have polycystic ovarian syndrome (PCOS).

CAUSES AND PREVENTION

There is no single cause for metabolic syndrome. There are multiple conditions that converge to create the syndrome. Some factors that result in metabolic syndrome include having a large waist, living a sedentary life, and insulin resistance. With increasing age, the risk of metabolic syndrome increases.

Q *Do I have a problem?*
Answer the questions below honestly.

1. Do you have an apple shape?   ☐ yes ☐ no
2. Do you have high levels of triglycerides?   ☐ yes ☐ no
3. Is your HDL cholesterol level less than 40?   ☐ yes ☐ no
4. Do you have high blood pressure?   ☐ yes ☐ no
5. Is your fasting blood sugar higher than normal?   ☐ yes ☐ no

You need to have a discussion with your health care provider about your answers. This is especially important if you answered "yes" to 3 or more of these questions. The more "yes" answers you gave, the greater your risk for heart disease, diabetes, and stroke.

Q *What can I do?*
If you have metabolic syndrome, then you have to control and manage all the underlying conditions. Regardless of whether or not you are diagnosed with metabolic syndrome, it is important to take the steps to enhance your health and life. Doing so not only will lengthen your life but will also improve your

quality of life. You need to revise your life goals and do whatever you can to reach them.

Stroke

Q *Que pasa?*
A stroke is a disease of the brain. Strokes are included in this section because too often a stroke is mistaken for a problem of the heart. When you have a stroke, the blood supply to your brain is interrupted either because there is blockage of a blood vessel supplying the brain (an ischemic stroke) or there is bleeding into or around the brain (a hemorrhagic stroke). The brain cells die when they no longer receive oxygen and nutrients from the blood.

CAUSES AND PREVENTION

The cause of strokes is unknown. There are 700,000 strokes in the United States every year. Strokes are less common among Hispanics than among non-Hispanic whites. People who smoke or have uncontrolled hypertension are likely to have a stroke.

Q *Do I have a problem?*
When looking at the symptoms of a stroke, the key word is *sudden*. Symptoms include sudden numbness or weakness, especially on one side of the body; sudden confusion or trouble speaking or understanding speech; sudden trouble seeing in one or both eyes; sudden trouble with walking, dizziness, or loss of balance or coordination; and sudden severe headache with no known cause.

Q *What can I do?*
Since quick action is essential, call 9-1-1 to get immediate help.

Sudden cardiac arrest

ALSO KNOWN AS
SCA _____

Q *Que pasa?*
All of a sudden your heart stops beating and the blood flow to your brain and the rest of your body stops. Death occurs within minutes. That is why most people who have SCA (95 percent) die. SCA is not a heart attack, although someone who has a heart attack may have an SCA while recovering from the heart attack.

CAUSES AND PREVENTION
SCAs tend to occur in people who seem healthy. They are usually individuals who are not considered at risk for heart disease. The diagnosis of SCA is made after the event and when other causes have been ruled out.

Q *Do I have a problem?*
The first sign of SCA is loss of consciousness and that the person has no heartbeat.

Q *What can I do?*
Since quick action is essential, you may want to familiarize yourself with how to use automated external defibrillators (AEDs). This equipment is increasingly found in easy-to-access

locations in airports, office buildings, shopping centers, other public places, and even some homes. These devices are programmed to give an electric shock if they detect a dangerous heart rhythm. They do not get activated if someone has only fainted.

Varicose veins

Q *Que pasa?*
Varicose veins appear when the valves in the vein are weak or damaged and the blood flows backward, creating pools that can cause that area to swell. These veins are right beneath the surface of the skin and can form anywhere in your body. They are usually found in your legs, but can also be found on the face and neck (called venous lakes), in the scrotum (called varicoceles), and behind the knees (flat blue veins called reticular veins). This common condition does not usually cause health problems. When they do, varicose veins cause pain, form blood clots, or lead to skin ulcers.

CAUSES AND PREVENTION
A family history of varicose veins, excess weight, pregnancy, getting older, being a woman, and staying in one position all the time are all factors that increase your risk of developing varicose veins. There is no way to prevent varicose veins from forming.

Q *Do I have a problem?*
Usually your health care provider will only need to do a physical exam to determine whether you have varicose veins. If you do, and they are severe, you may be referred to a vascular medicine specialist or a vascular surgeon for further care.

Q *What can I do?*
To reduce the pain and discomfort from varicose veins, here are some steps you can take:

1. Stay active. If you have to stand or sit for long periods, make sure you take regular breaks and move around. Raise your legs when sitting, resting, or sleeping. As often as you can, keep your legs above the level of your heart.
2. Keep your legs moving as much as possible. This helps to build and strengthen the muscles in your legs. Avoid crossing your legs.
3. Maintain a healthy weight to reduce the pressure on your veins.
4. Wear loose clothing. Clothing that is tight, especially around your waist, groin (upper thighs), and legs, can make varicose veins worse.
5. Wear lower-heeled shoes. They tone your calf muscles and help blood move through the veins. Shoes with high heels are bad for your veins and bad for your feet.

Vasculitis

ALSO KNOWN AS
angiitis or arteritis

Q *Que pasa?*
This is when any of the arteries, veins, or capillaries get inflamed and narrow as a result. In serious cases, the narrowing of the blood vessel can be so severe as to completely close it off. Vasculitis may affect specific large, medium, or small blood vessels; your overall body (known as systemic vasculitis); your brain and spinal cord; or specific organs.

CAUSES AND PREVENTION

It is not known what causes the blood vessels to get inflamed. For some unknown reason, the immune system in the body becomes engaged to attack the blood vessels because they are mistakenly perceived as an invading substance. The immune system may be triggered due to an ongoing infection; an autoimmune disease that a person has, such as lupus or rheumatoid arthritis; or in reaction to medication.

People who smoke or who have chronic hepatitis B or C, lupus, or another autoimmune disease have a higher risk of vasculitis. There is no known way to prevent vasculitis.

Q *Do I have a problem?*
If you have vasculitis, you will experience symptoms that are common with inflammation, such as fever and general aches and pains. Some people have very few symptoms while others become very ill. What will determine your symptoms and how well you do with treatment is whether the vasculitis is in your skin, joints, lungs, gastrointestinal tract, sinuses, nose, ear, throat, ears, eyes, brain, or nerves. In most cases, treatment is successful.

Q *What can I do?*
The type of vasculitis you have determines what changes you have to make in your life. Sometimes with medications the vasculitis will go away and never come back. In the beginning you will need close monitoring by your health care provider because the medicines that are given are very strong. As with any chronic condition, the support of family and friends makes it easier to manage what may be a lifelong condition.

Diagnostic tests and procedures

While your health care provider will give you written and verbal instructions on how to prepare for your test or procedures, here are some facts to help you better understand what will be happening. Remember it is your responsibility to ask your health care provider for another explanation if you do not understand what you are being told.

Cardiac catheterization

Q What is this?
This procedure is used to diagnose and treat the heart. In most cases, the procedure is done in the hospital in the cardiac catheterization laboratory, also known as the "cath lab."

During cardiac catheterization, you are awake but sleepy and there is very little, if any, pain. The person doing the procedure shaves and numbs the area where the catheter—a long, very thin, flexible tube—will be inserted (usually in your arm, upper thigh, or neck). The catheter is then inserted into your coronary artery and carefully moved toward your heart. Using x-ray images, your health care provider is able to look at the arteries in your heart, check the pressure and blood flow in your heart's chambers, and collect blood samples. Sometimes a dye is injected into your coronary arteries or your heart chambers so that the flow of blood is easier to follow. The catheter allows your cardiologist to use small instruments to take samples of the heart muscle and even to do some minor procedures.

Q *What can I expect?*

You will need to rest after the procedure. You will probably have a small bruise where the catheter was inserted. The area will be sore for a week. Talk to your cardiologist and ask if there are activities you should avoid.

Q *Are there risks?*

Death is rare with cardiac catheterization. There are increased risks of complications for women, people with diabetes or kidney disease, people over 75 years old, and when the procedure is done on an emergency basis.

Cardiac CT

ALSO KNOWN AS
computed tomography, coronary artery scan, coronary CT angiography, computed tomographic coronary angiography, or CTCA, and heart CT scan

---

Q *What is this?*

In computed tomography (CT), multiple x-rays are taken and then put together by a computer to generate a detailed 3D (3-dimensional) image of your internal organs. Cardiac CT shows the size and shape of the heart and is much more detailed than ultrasound. In some cases a dye may be injected into your veins to highlight the blood vessels and give a clearer image.

Q What can I expect?
The procedure will be done in a hospital or in the offices of your health care provider. You may have an iodine-based dye injected into one of your veins during the scan or before you take the test. Be sure to let your health care provider know if you have allergies to any medicines, iodine, or shellfish. You will probably be given medicines to slow down your heart (beta blockers) so that the images taken are better. Although the actual procedure takes only 15 minutes, it can take an hour to do all the preparations.

Q Are there risks?
During the procedure you will be exposed to an amount of radiation that is equal to the total amount that you would naturally be exposed to in a 3-year period. The amount of radiation involved creates a greater cancer risk for people under 40.

Cardiac MRI

ALSO KNOWN AS
heart MRI, cardiovascular MRI, cardiac nuclear magnetic
resonance, or NMR, and MRI scan

What is this?

In an MRI (magnetic resonance imaging), magnets and radio waves are used to create images that give precise information about the location and size of whatever is being imaged. The images that are produced in a cardiac MRI include pictures of your heart when it is still and when it is moving. The moving pictures help your health care provider see how the heart is working. Cardiac MRI also helps explain results from tests that use x-rays, such as cardiac CT scans.

What can I expect?

The test will be done in a hospital or at an imaging center. This procedure will take from 45 to 90 minutes.

Are there risks?

This common procedure is considered a painless and harmless way to get information on how the heart works. If the MRI includes a stress test, then there may be side effects from any additional medication that is given as part of the stress test. If you have an implanted pacemaker or defibrillator, you cannot have an MRI because it may make your implanted device malfunction. All the existing evidence indicates that neither the magnets nor the radio waves result in any side effects.

Carotid endarterectomy

ALSO KNOWN AS
CEA and carotid artery procedure

> I kept getting headaches that did not go away but I
> had to go to work and so willed them away. What
> alternative did I have? There was no sense in trying to
> get help, since every health care provider I saw said
> that there was nothing wrong. I was told it was prob-
> ably menopause or malaise. Finally, I found a health
> care provider who listened to me. Before I knew it, I
> was having procedure to clear a blockage. —Rebecca

What is this?

This surgical procedure removes plaque from the two large arteries on either side of your neck. It is believed that it reduces the risk of stroke in people who have carotid artery disease (see "Atherosclerosis," page 53). There are also medicines to treat carotid artery disease.

What can I expect?

You should have a serious discussion with your health care provider as to whether this procedure is necessary. Complications from CEA are more likely in women and in people over 75 who have other risk factors. Be aware that, although uncommon, there is a small risk that during or after this procedure you will have a stroke. The procedure is usually done in the hospital and takes about 2 hours. Most people stay in the hospital for 1 or 2 days and return to their regular routine in 3 weeks.

Carotid ultrasound imaging

ALSO KNOWN AS
Doppler ultrasound and carotid duplex ultrasound

Q *What is this?*
In this test, high-frequency sound waves (ultrasound) are used to create an image of the large arteries on each side of your neck (the carotid arteries) that supply blood to your brain. The images show if the arteries have narrowed. It is usually recommended if you have had a stroke or a ministroke or if your health care provider hears an abnormal sound in your carotid artery.

Q *What can I expect?*
This is a painless and harmless test that is usually done in the office of your health care provider or in a hospital. It takes about 30 minutes.

Coronary angiography

Q *What is this?*
This is when cardiac catheterization, x-rays, and sometimes special dyes are used to produce images of the insides of arteries, including the amount of damage and blockage to blood vessels. These images are taken during cardiac catheterization, which is an invasive procedure that has some risks. Sometimes angiography and coronary angioplasty are done at the same time.

Q **What can I expect?**
Based on the images that are developed, your cardiologist will have more information to share with you about the type of heart problem that you have. Complications from this procedure are more likely to occur in women, people over 75 years old, people who have diabetes or kidney disease, and people who are having the procedure on an emergency basis. Fatal complications are rare.

Coronary angioplasty

ALSO KNOWN AS
balloon angioplasty, coronary artery angioplasty, invasive coronary angioplasty, or ICA, and percutaneous coronary intervention, or PCI

Q **What is this?**
This is a procedure that widens blocked arteries. A cardiologist in a hospital catheterization laboratory performs it. Coronary angioplasty is one of the procedures that can be done through cardiac catheterization. A small mesh tube, called a *stent,* is wrapped around the deflated balloon catheter before the catheter is inserted in the artery. The stent is guided to the area where there is blockage. Once there, the balloon is inflated to compress the plaque. The stent then expands and becomes attached to the artery wall. In this way, the stent supports the inner artery wall and reduces the chance of the artery becoming narrowed or blocked again. Some stents are coated with medications that are slowly and continuously released into the artery. *Carotid angioplasty* refers to a similar procedure that is used to eliminate blockages in the carotid arteries.

Q ***What can I expect?***
You will fast before the procedure and be given other instructions by your cardiologist. The procedure will take about 1 to 2 hours. Throughout the procedure you will be awake, although you will be very calm because of the medications that you are getting intravenously (by IV) to relax you. Most people stay in the hospital at least one night.

Q ***What are the risks?***
Each year 1 million people in the United States undergo angioplasty. Less than 2 percent of people die from angioplasty. Complications are more likely for people over 75 years old, persons with kidney disease or diabetes, women, people with hearts that have problems pumping, and people who have extensive heart disease or blockages.

Coronary artery bypass grafting

ALSO KNOWN AS
CABG, bypass procedure, coronary artery bypass procedure, and heart bypass procedure

Q ***What is this?***
In this type of procedure, a surgeon removes a healthy artery or vein from one part of the body and reconnects it to bypass a blocked artery. There are several types of CABG procedures: traditional CABG, off-pump CABG, port-access coronary artery bypass procedure, minimally invasive direct coronary artery bypass (MIDCAB) grafting, and robot-assisted technique. In traditional CABG, the heart is stopped and a heart-lung bypass machine is used to pump blood and oxygen to the body. In off-pump CABG, or beating heart bypass graft, since the heart is not stopped, there

is no need for a heart-lung bypass machine. With the port-access coronary artery bypass procedure, small incisions are made in your chest and a heart-lung bypass machine is used. In MIDCAB grafting, the surgeon makes small incisions on the left side of the chest between the ribs. This relatively new procedure is used to bypass blood vessels in the front of the heart. Robot-assisted techniques use keyhole-sized incisions that are remotely controlled by a surgeon. Sometimes a heart-lung bypass machine is used.

Your cardiologist will decide whether or not you are a good candidate for this procedure. The recommendation to have this procedure will take into account the severity and location of blockages, your age, your response to other treatments and lifestyle changes, and the consequences of other health problems that you have.

What can I expect?

Q This procedure is done in the hospital under general anesthesia and takes 3 to 5 hours. When you come out of the recovery room, you spend 1 to 2 days in the intensive care unit (ICU), followed by 3 to 5 days in the hospital before you go home. When you go home, you will be given extensive written and verbal instructions on how to take care of yourself. The longest recovery time is after traditional CABG; following that procedure, full recovery takes 6 to 12 weeks. Talk to your health care provider about when you can resume sexual activity (usually within 4 weeks), driving (after 3 to 8 weeks), and your other everyday activities.

The risk of complications from any of the CABG procedures is greater for women; if the procedure is done in an emergency situation; for people over 70 years of age, for smokers, and for people with diabetes, kidney disease, lung disease, or peripheral arterial disease.

Echocardiography

ALSO KNOWN AS
echo, surface echo, and ultrasound of the heart

Q *What is this?*
This procedure creates images of the heart using sound waves. Echoes do not involve an invasive procedure or exposure to x-rays. The images that are generated show the size and shape of the heart. They can also show if there are problems in the functioning of the chambers and valves in the heart, the presence of blood clots or tumors, the buildup of fluid, and problems with the aorta. A Doppler ultrasound echo also gives information on the flow of blood through the chambers and valves of your heart.

There are different types of echoes. Some of the echos involve putting a device on your chest (transthoracic echocardiography), taking images as you exercise and as you rest (stress echocardiography), or taking images from a tiny tube that is guided through your throat and into your esophagus (transesophageal echocardiography or TEE). Images from a transthoracic or TEE may be combined to create a 3D image of the heart (3-dimensional echocardiography).

Q *What can I expect?*
This is a painless and harmless test that is usually done in the office of your cardiologist or in a hospital. Depending on the type of echo ordered for you, you may have to make some special preparations. For example, if you are going to have a TEE, you will be asked not to drink or eat anything for 8 hours before the test. It takes about 30 minutes.

Electrocardiogram

ALSO KNOWN AS
EKG, ECG, 12-lead EKG, and 12-lead ECG

Q ***What is this?***
This test records the heart's electrical activity—how fast is it beating and whether the rhythm is steady or irregular. It also records the strength and frequency of the electrical signals. Your health care provider may use the results as one measure of whether you have had or are having a heart attack and the extent of damage to your heart. It is also one way that your health care provider may be able to detect heart disease before you experience symptoms. An EKG also gives valuable information about the blood flow to the heart muscle, whether the heart can pump forcefully, whether the heart muscle is too thick or has become enlarged, whether there are problems with heart valves, and other conditions.

Q ***What can I expect?***
Depending on your age and health history, an EKG may be part of your routine physical exam. For this 10-minute test, you will have to take off your shirt and pants as soft sticky patches with wires attached, called electrodes, are placed on your chest, arms, and legs to pick up the electrical signals that your body gives off.

Heart surgery

Q ***What is this?***
This includes all procedures to improve the functioning of the heart, from the most common (coronary artery bypass procedure, or CABG) to heart valve repair or replacement to a heart transplant. Open-heart surgery is where the surgeon opens the chest to do the procedure. It is becoming more common to do off-pump open-heart surgery, that is, not use a heart-lung bypass machine.

Q ***What can I expect?***
In most cases the risks of complications from heart surgery are greater for women and people who are over 70 or have high blood pressure, diabetes, kidney disease, lung disease, or peripheral arterial disease. With each heart surgery, the risk for complications also increases.

Heart transplant

Q ***What is this?***
This is surgery to replace a heart that will not work much longer with a healthy heart from a deceased person. The need for this surgery is less than had been projected, as many heart problems can be treated because of the scientific advances in early diagnosis and intervention, medication, angioplasty, and other procedures.

Q What can I expect?
Most patients (72 percent) survive for 5 years and 50 percent survive for 10 years. Although most (60 percent) do
not return to work, the majority (90 percent) report that they
come close to resuming their previous life.

Holter monitors and event monitors

ALSO KNOWN AS
ambulatory EKG or ECG, continuous EKG, EKG event monitors, episodic monitors, mobile cardiac outpatient teleme-
try systems, autodetect recorders, 30-day event recorders,
and transtelephonic event monitors

Q What is this?
These monitors are devices that record the electrical activity of the heart. They are used to track how the heart is
working when the person has no symptoms but other factors
suggest that there are problems with the electrical activity of the
heart, such as fainting or feeling dizzy or experiencing palpitations in your chest, throat, or neck.

There are different kinds of monitors. A Holter monitor will
record the electrical activity of your heart on a nonstop basis as
you go through your day. It is about the size of a deck of cards.
For the 24 to 48 hours you use it, you will only be able to take a
sponge bath. Wireless Holter monitors can be worn for longer
periods, and you can detach the sensors to shower. Information is
continuously sent to your health care provider or to a company
that monitors the data that are transmitted. An event monitor is a

slightly smaller device that does not monitor continuously; it only records electrical activities when you push a button to indicate that you are having symptoms. Autodetect recorders are designed to record automatically when unusual heart rhythms are picked up. For all monitors, small patches with electrodes are attached to your chest with a body paste. These electrodes are connected to a small, portable recorder. In all cases you wear the monitor clipped to a belt, in a pocket, or around your neck as you go about your usual routine. Postevent recorders have neither wires nor sensors. They are either worn like a wristwatch or you can use another version that is the size of thick credit card. When you feel you are having a symptom, you turn on the device and hold it to your chest to record the data. The data are stored and you can send it to your health care provider over the telephone or via the Internet. Implantable loop recorders are more invasive because the monitor is inserted under the skin in your chest.

Q What can I expect?
In addition to wearing the monitor, you will be asked to keep a journal of your activities and of any symptoms you experience. Your results may help your health care provider determine whether or not you have a problem.

Implantable cardioverter defibrillator

ALSO KNOWN AS
ICD

Q *What is this?*

This device is implanted in your chest to help you have regular heartbeats and to prevent sudden cardiac arrest (SCA). The ICD is a little metal box that has a battery, a pulse generator, and a computer. It also has one wire (single-chamber ICDs) or more wires (dual-chamber ICDs) that connect the computer to the chamber or chambers in your heart. The electrical signals in your heart are tracked by the ICD so that, when necessary, the ICD can send back low-energy pulses to correct the rhythm. In more urgent cases, the defibrillator will be activated and send a high-energy electrical pulse (shock).

Q *What can I expect?*

It takes only a few hours to implant the ICD. You will have to be careful about how long you are in contact with electrical devices or are close to strong magnetic fields, which means you cannot have an MRI. There are many devices that can disrupt your ICD: for example, cell phones, iPods, household appliances, microwave ovens, high-tension power lines, metal detectors, industrial welders, and electrical generators. Regular communication with your health care provider will be particularly important.

Nuclear heart scan

ALSO KNOWN AS

nuclear stress test, SPECT scan, or single positron emission computed tomography scan, and PET scan, or positron emission tomography scan

***

Q *What is this?*

These tests create a picture of how well blood is flowing through your heart muscle and how much blood is reaching your heart muscle. In these tests you are injected with a radioactive substance called a tracer. The substances that are used are considered safe, and there have been no reports of negative long-term effects. Once your vein has been injected with the tracer, it is given time to travel to your heart, where it releases energy. The release of energy by the tracer is recorded by special cameras outside the body. The recordings are used to create pictures of your heart. A nuclear heart scan can show the location and extent of damage in the heart.

SPECT and PET scans use different tracers. SPECT scans have been used for a while and show problems with blood flow, damaged or dead heart tissue, and how the lower-left chamber pumps blood to the body. A PET scan is a newer type of scan that provides a more detailed and clearer picture. At this point there is no clear advantage for either one.

Q *What can I expect?*

This will probably be done in a hospital. It will take 2 to 5 hours to complete a scan. The results of your scan will help your health care provider and cardiologist diagnose and manage your heart disease, have a better idea of your risk of having a heart attack, and decide which are the best treatment options for you.

Pacemaker

Q What is this?

This small device is implanted in your chest to track and help control your heartbeat. A pacemaker is a thin metal box that has a battery, a generator with a computer, and multiple wires with sensors. The sensors detect your heart rhythm. The latest models have sensors that also track your blood temperature, breathing, and other factors related to your activity. Pacemakers can be single-chamber, dual-chamber, or biventricular. There are 2 types of pacemakers: demand and rate-responsive. The demand pacemaker only sends a signal if there is an irregularity in the heartbeat. The rate-responsive pacemaker monitors several factors to determine your activity and then make sure that the heart is beating at the desired rate.

Q What can I expect?

You will have surgery to have the pacemaker implanted in a hospital and stay at least 1 night. The risk of any problem is very low. It will be best for you to take it easy for a few days, and then you will be able to return to your daily activities. The major change is that you will have to be careful about being close to electrical devices for long periods and you will also have to avoid strong magnetic fields, which means you cannot have an MRI. You will have to follow special precautions when using or being close to cell phones, iPods, household appliances, microwave ovens, high-tension power lines, metal detectors, industrial welders, and electrical generators.

Stress testing

ALSO KNOWN AS

exercise echocardiogram or exercise stress echo, exercise test, myocardial perfusion imaging, nuclear stress test, PET stress test, pharmacological stress test, sestamibi stress test, stress EKG, thallium stress test, and treadmill test

Q What is this?

The purpose of this test is to see how your heart functions when it is stressed. As part of this test you are physically stressed by either being given exercises to do (walking or running on a treadmill or pedaling a bicycle) or medicines to make your heart work harder while the tests are done. The goal is to see how your heart works when it needs more oxygen and blood. Images of your heart are made while you are at rest and at full exertion. The stress test is used in combination with one of the many diagnostic or imaging procedures that are used.

Q What can I expect?

This is not a routine screening test for heart problems. The results of this test are more meaningful for men than for women. Research has shown that for one-third of women, the results of stress tests are not as accurate as they are for men. The images that are taken during the test help to identify if there are problems with the flow of blood in and out of your heart. In 1 in 5,000 people, the stress test itself can cause a heart attack or death.

Part Three

RESOURCES AND TOOLS TO HELP YOU TAKE CONTROL

If you have questions about your heart, please call the National Hispanic Family Health Help Line at 866-783-2645, or 866-Su-Familia. Health promotion advisors are available to answer your questions in English and Spanish and help you find local services. You can call Monday through Friday, from 9 A.M. to 6 P.M. EST.

BEST NONCOMMERCIAL WEBSITES

AMERICAN COLLEGE OF CARDIOLOGY
www.cardiosmart.org

AMERICAN HEART ASSOCIATION
www.americanheart.org

NATIONAL ALLIANCE FOR HISPANIC HEALTH
hispanichealth.org

NATIONAL HEART, LUNG, AND BLOOD INSTITUTE (NHLBI)
www.nhlbi.nih.gov

NATIONAL INSTITUTE OF NEUROLOGICAL DISORDERS AND STROKE
www.ninds.nih.gov

NATIONAL LIBRARY OF MEDICINE (NLM): MEDLINEPLUS
www.nlm.nih.gov

ABOUT ME

MY BLOOD TYPE_____ **ALLERGIES**_____

Date	Blood Pressure	Weight	HDL	LDL	Total Cholesterol	Triglycerides	Urine	Other
	/							
	/							
	/							
	/							
	/							
	/							
	/							
	/							
	/							
	/							
	/							
	/							
	/							
	/							
	/							
	/							

VISITS TO MY HEALTH CARE PROVIDER

DATE _____ WHY I WENT _____
_____

WHOM I SAW _____
_____

SPECIAL TESTS _____
_____

DIAGNOSIS _____
_____

REFERRED ELSEWHERE _____
_____

MEDICINES PRESCRIBED _____
_____

WHAT ELSE DID THE HEALTH CARE PROVIDER DO/SAY? _____
_____
_____
_____

DATE _____ WHY I WENT _____
_____

WHOM I SAW _____
_____

SPECIAL TESTS _____
_____

DIAGNOSIS _____
_____

REFERRED ELSEWHERE _____
_____

MEDICINES PRESCRIBED _____
_____

WHAT ELSE DID THE HEALTH CARE PROVIDER DO/SAY? _____
_____
_____
_____

My Medicines, Vitamins, Supplements, Teas, and Other Things I Take

NAME _____ COST _____

PURPOSE _____

SIZE/AMOUNT _____ COLOR _____ SHAPE _____

DATE PRESCRIBED _____ BY _____

HOW MUCH DO I TAKE? _____ WHEN? _____

THINGS TO AVOID _____

SIDE EFFECTS/OTHER COMMENTS _____

_____

_____

_____

NAME _____ COST _____

PURPOSE _____

SIZE/AMOUNT _____ COLOR _____ SHAPE _____

DATE PRESCRIBED _____ BY _____

HOW MUCH DO I TAKE? _____ WHEN? _____

THINGS TO AVOID _____

SIDE EFFECTS/OTHER COMMENTS _____

_____

_____

_____

QUESTIONS TO DISCUSS WITH YOUR HEALTH CARE PROVIDER

QUESTIONS TO ASK ABOUT A DIAGNOSIS

1. *Can you please repeat that?*

2. *What does that mean?*

3. *Could you draw me a picture?*

4. *How does that change what I have to do?*

5. *What will I do next?*

QUESTIONS TO ASK ABOUT A DIAGNOSTIC TEST

1. *Can you please repeat the name of the test?*

2. *What will the test show?*

3. *Where will I have the test?*

4. *Are there any risks involved?*

5. *What special preparations should I make before the test?*

6. *How long will it take?*

7. *What will happen after the test?*

8. *Is there anything else I should know?*

9. *Who will give me the results?*

10. *How long will it take to get the results?*

QUESTIONS TO ASK ABOUT SURGERY OR PROCEDURES

1. *Do I have to have surgery, or are there any nonsurgical options?*

2. *What would you expect to be different for me if I have this surgery?*

3. *Have there been problems with this type of surgery?*

4. *How successful is this surgery?*

5. *Which hospital is best for this surgery?*

6. *Where can I get a second opinion about the surgery I am considering?*

7. *If I go with your recommendation, who will actually be doing the surgery? If it is someone other than you, when will I meet that person?*

8. *How many times have you (or that person) done this surgery?*

9. *I know there are different kinds of anesthesia. Can you explain how they differ and which one you think would be best for me?*

10. *I know it is important to meet the anesthesiologist before my surgery. When will I meet her or him?*

11. *How long will the actual surgery take?*

12. *Will the person I designate as my health care advocate be kept informed about the progress of my surgery while it is under way and, afterward, the result of the surgery?*

13. *Whom can I ask whether my health insurance will cover all aspects of the surgery—the pre–hospital admission tests, the hospital stay, the surgeons and anesthesiologists, the rehabilitative services, and so on?*

QUESTIONS TO ASK ABOUT RECOVERY
AFTER SURGERY OR PROCEDURES

1. *How long after the surgery will I have to stay in the hospital?*

2. *After the surgery, how much pain will I have?*

3. *Will I be given medicines to take at home?*

4. *Will I be able to go home after the surgery, or will I probably need additional care elsewhere? If I cannot go directly home, where will I go, and when will I be able to go home?*

5. *Will I be able to drive home? If not, how long will it be before I can drive?*

6. *When I go home, will I need*
   - *Someone to help me with my daily activities?* Yes   No
   - *Special food?* Yes   No
   - *Special equipment?* Yes   No

7. *When I am home, will I be able to*
   - *Go to the bathroom by myself?* Yes   No (If no, when can I?)
   - *Shower by myself?* Yes   No (if no, when)
   - *Go up and down stairs?* Yes   No (if no, when)
   - *Cook for myself?* Yes   No (if no, when)

8. *How soon after surgery will I be able to return to my daily routine?*

9. *When will I need to have follow-up appointments? Will those be with you or with someone else?*

⌒Acknowledgments

There are many people who make the *Buena Salud*™ series possible. The entire team at Newmarket Press, especially Esther Margolis, Heidi Sachner, Keith Hollaman, and Harry Burton, have pro-vided incredible encouragement. The board, staff, and members of the National Alliance for Hispanic Health and the Health Foundation for the Americas also nurtured the creation of the series. For this edition, John C. (Jack) Lewin, M.D., internist, and Hector O. Ventura, M.D., internist and cardiologist, volunteered their time and experience to make sure that the *Guide* was up-to-date and accurate.

The personal support that I need to write came from my life sisters and brothers as well as exceptional friends and include Kevin Adams, Carolyn Curiel, Msgr. Duffy, Adolph P. Falcón, Polly Gault, Paula Gomez, Ileana Herrell, Thomas Pheasant, Sheila Raviv, Carolina Reyes, Esther Sciammarella, Cynthia A. Telles, and Elizabeth Valdez. My memories and experiences with my extraordinary mother, Lucy Delgado, my cousin Deborah Helvarg, and my friend Henrietta Villaescusa are also part of this book.

Most of all I want to thank my husband, Mark, and daughter, Elizabeth, for the inspiration and affection they provide on a daily basis. Their love frames my life and gives me the emotional sustenance for everything I do.

INDEX

ABOUT THE AUTHOR

JANE L. DELGADO, Ph.D., M.S., author of *The Latina Guide to Health: Consejos and Caring Answers*, is President and Chief Executive Officer of the National Alliance for Hispanic Health ("the Alliance"), the nation's largest organization of health and human service providers to Hispanics. She was recognized by the *Ladies' Home Journal* as one of the "Ladies We Love" in 2010 and by *WebMD* as one of its four Health Heroes of 2008 for her dedication and resilience in advocacy. Among many other awards and honors, in 2007 *People En Español* named her to the 100 Influentials in the Hemisphere.

A practicing clinical psychologist, Dr. Delgado joined the Alliance in 1985 after serving in the Immediate Office of the Secretary of the U.S. Department of Health and Human Services (DHHS), where she became a key force in the development of the landmark "Report of the Secretary's Task Force on Black and Minority Health."

At the Alliance, Dr. Delgado oversees the national staff as well as field operations throughout the United States, Puerto Rico, and the District of Columbia. She is also a trustee of the Kresge Foundation, Lovelace Respiratory Research Institute, the U.S. Soccer Foundation, Northern Virginia Health Foundation, and the Health Foundation for the Americas, and serves on the national advisory councils for the Paul G. Rogers Society for Global Health Research and on the National Board of Mrs. Rosalyn Carter's Task Force on Mental Health.

Dr. Delgado received her M.A. in Psychology from New York University in 1975. In 1981 she was awarded a Ph.D. in clinical psychology from SUNY Stony Brook and an M.S. in Urban and Policy Sciences from the W. Averell Harriman School of Urban and Policy Sciences. She lives in Washington, D.C., with her husband, Mark, and daughter, Elizabeth.

Founded in 1973, the **National Alliance for Hispanic Health** is the foremost science-based source of information and trusted advocate for the health of Hispanics. The Alliance represents local community agencies serving more than 15 million persons each year, and national organizations serving over 100 million persons, making a daily difference in the lives of Hispanic communities and families.

The **Health Foundation for the Americas (HFA)** supports the work and mission of the National Alliance for Hispanic Health, and seeks individuals, companies, agencies, foundations, and sponsors to help support its programs to improve the quality of healthcare for all, which includes providing timely and trusted bilingual health information. Every year HFA supports programs to improve health for all by helping secure clean air to breathe, clean water to drink, safe places to play, and healthy food to eat. HFA and the Alliance help those without healthcare gain access to free and low-cost services where they live and improve the quality of healthcare. The programs put new health technology to work in communities, provide millions of dollars in science and health career scholarships, and conduct the research and advocacy that is transforming health.

Dr. Delgado's book *The Latina Guide to Health: Consejos and Caring Answers* is published simultaneously in English- and Spanish-language editions by Newmarket Press. The author is donating all royalties from the Spanish edition to The Health Foundation for the Americas (HFA).

You can be a part of this extraordinary mission of health and well-being. To learn more about the Alliance or the HFA, visit www.hispanichealth.org or www.healthyamericas.org.

Newmarket Titles by Jane L. Delgado

Written specifically for the growing U.S. Latino population by Jane L. Delgado, Ph.D., M.S., the president and CEO of the National Alliance for Hispanic Health, *The Buena Salud™ Guides* present the best in health advice, available in both English and Spanish-language editions.

The Buena Salud™ Guide to Diabetes and Your Life
Introduction by Larry Hausner, CEO, America Diabetes Association

Featuring the stories of people and families living with diabetes—a condition that has touched the lives of most Hispanic families—this concise guide explains everything readers need to know, including the important fact that diabetes is not inevitable.

    The book discusses: the factors that contribute to developing diabetes and how to prevent it; the types and evolving definition of diabetes; how the endocrine and immune systems function; the impact of the environment on diabetes; treatment options, including medication and realistic changes in lifestyle and diet; and features an A-Z section with all commonly used diabetes terms.

Paperback • 128 pages • ISBN: 978-1-55704-941-4 • $9.95

Also available in Spanish:
La guía de Buena Salud™ sobre la diabetes y tu vida (978-1-55704-942-1)

The Buena Salud™ Guide for a Healthy Heart
Introduction by Jack Lewin, M.D., CEO, American College of Cardiology

Opening with a personal story from Dr. Delgado about her mother's experience with heart disease, this invaluable guide details everything readers need to know about the leading cause of death for all men and women in the U.S.

    The book explains: how the heart works; how heart problems develop and what can be done to avoid them; achievable lifestyle changes to maintain heart health; and features an A-Z section with all commonly used heart terms.

Paperback • 128 pages • ISBN: 978-1-55704-943-8 • $9.95

Also available in Spanish:
La guía de Buena Salud™ para un corazón sano (978-1-55704-944-5)

Thunder from the Mountains

Edited by Maina wa Kinyatti

Dedicated to —

The Youth of Kenya on whom the future of
our country now depends.

And all those who struggled and sacrificed
for the liberation of our country from
British colonialism.

Thunder from the Mountains
Mau Mau Patriotic Songs

Edited by Maina wa Kinyatti

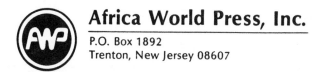

Africa World Press, Inc.

P.O. Box 1892
Trenton, New Jersey 08607

Africa World Press, Inc
P.O. Box 1892
Trenton, NJ 08607

Copyright (c) 1990 by Maina wa Kinyatti,

First Africa World Press, Inc. Edition 1990

First published by Zed Press and Midi-Tiki, 1980

Cover design by Ife Nii Owoo

ISBN: 0-86543-204-X HB
       0-86543-205-8 PB

Contents

Acknowledgements

In collecting these songs I spent many days and nights in the homes of former Mau Mau guerrillas, peasants and workers, recording their voices as they sang. Many thanks are due to them.

My sincere thanks are also due to Kinuthia wa Mugia, Muthee wa Cheche, Gakaara wa Wanjau, J.M. Kariuki, Karari wa Njama and Mohamed Mathu who wrote, edited and compiled some of these songs.

Finally, I would like to point out that the translation of these songs is the result of a collective effort on the part of many individuals whose comments and suggestions I have freely incorporated in this work. Needless to say, the final responsibility in translation lies with me, but the views expressed in the songs are entirely those of the thousands and thousands of Kenyans who, because of their patriotism, joined the struggle against the British colonial occupiers.

Acknowledgements

In collecting these songs I spent many days and nights in the homes of former Mau Mau guerrillas, peasants and workers, recording their voices as they sang. Many thanks are due to them.

My sincere thanks are also due to Kinuthia wa Mugia, Muthee wa Cheche, Gakaara wa Wanjau, J.M. Kariuki, Karari wa Njama and Mohamed Mathu who wrote, edited and compiled some of these songs.

Finally, I would like to point out that the translation of these songs is the result of a collective effort on the part of many individuals whose comments and suggestions I have freely incorporated in this work. Needless to say, the final responsibility in translation lies with me, but the views expressed in the songs are entirely those of the thousands and thousands of Kenyans who, because of their patriotism, joined the struggle against the British colonial occupiers.

Preface

Within a span of five years Mau Mau produced most formidable political songs which the Movement used as a weapon to politicize and educate the Kenyan worker and peasant masses. This helped heighten the people's consciousness against the forces of the foreign occupiers and, in the process, prepared them for armed struggle. The role of these songs in educating the workers and peasants against the dictatorship of the colonialists was an undeniable catalyst in the development and success of the Movement.

These songs were sung at Kenya African Union (KAU) rallies, in Independent Schools and churches, in the homes of the ordinary people, in guerrilla bases, in detention camps and in prisons. In essence, the songs urged the entire oppressed population of Kenya to take up arms and expel British colonialism from the country. Some of the songs particularly called upon the patriotic petty-bourgeois elements to support the workers and peasants against the foreign enemy and its local allies. They also taught the people to differentiate between friends and enemies, to understand thoroughly the designs and intentions of the enemy, and, quite importantly, to know that true freedom is not something that can just be given or donated without struggle by the masses. It must be fought for at great sacrifice. The songs tried to answer the fundamental questions in a colony: What is patriotism? And therefore, who are patriots and who are traitors? Fundamentally, these were class distinctions of great subsequent political importance in Kenya.

These songs are a monumental testimony to the greatness of the Mau Mau movement. They also provide important information which enables us to become more familiar with the political goals and heroism of Mau Mau.

The songs reproduced here are arranged chronologically. Part One consists of the mass songs which were composed before the British declared war on our people on October 20, 1952. These songs were used by the Movement to politicize and educate the general population about the nature of British colonialism in order to win their support for armed struggle. They express our people's hatred of the colonialists and their local 'boys'. The major themes running through them are the demands of the people for the return of their stolen land and for freedom and recognition of their dignity, and culture as a nation.

Part Two is composed of detention and prison songs from the early war years. They highlight the suffering in the camps and prisons. They express the people's bitterness against the 'Home Guard' traitors who were hunting, spying on and torturing them in the camps and who superintended their eviction from the settlers' plantations. The songs make it clear to these traitors that they will pay with their lives for such treachery. Some of them also eulogize the Mau Mau guerrillas in the forests for their heroism and express their confidence and faith in Field Marshall Dedan Kimathi's leadership. Finally, they articulate the people's optimism that they will win the struggle against the forces of the occupation. Politically, the songs in this section seem clearer than those in Part One.

Part Three is comprised of lyrics by guerrillas. One can sense the very flames of war in them. They glorify the revolutionary aspects of the Movement: its dialectical relationship with the worker and peasant masses on the one hand, and its principled contradiction with British colonialism on the other. They again praise the heroism of the guerrillas and their leaders. They tell stories of outstanding battles fought by the Mau Mau forces; they speak of the patriotism of the women and youth and the great sacrifices they had to make in support of, and for participating in, the fighting. At the same time the lyrics articulate the guerrillas' deep hatred for British colonialism. They often point out that both these foreign occupiers and the local traitors should be regarded as Kenya's enemy number one who should be wiped out mercilessly. There runs through the songs a consistent spirit of optimism that the people of Kenya and their Mau Mau army will, in the end, win the war. The content of these lyrics is patriotic, anti-colonial and anti-imperialist.

In summary, the main objective in translating these songs is to let them answer the anti-Mau Mau Kenyan intellectuals and their imperialist masters who, until now, continue to deny the Movement's national character.

Maina wa Kinyatti
Nairobi, Kenya
1979

Introduction

It is difficult for those Kenyans who were born after the mid 1950s to realize the bitter suffering that our people experienced during the subjugation of our country by British colonialism from 1888 to 1963. People were forced to live like beggars and tramps in the land of their birth, and many patriots were murdered outright when they resisted the imperialists occupying our country.

This was the darkest period of our history: the period of foreign domination, unbearable colonial exploitation, the calculated massacre of the Kenyan people, and systematic destruction of our national cultures. We learn from Amilcar Cabral that 'to take up arms to dominate a people, is, above all, to take up arms to destroy its cultural life.'[1] Similarly, the British colonialists used brutal cultural repression in order to reduce us to slavery. With complete control of the mass media and schools, the colonialists made full use of them to distort and crush our national cultures and history, and thereby to suppress our patriotic feelings. In the process this involved attempting to shape our political outlook and promoting a cult of British capitalist culture.

In schools our children were subjected to the worst form of brainwashing. They were taught that the British imperialists were 'generous liberators' of our country from the Arab slavers, and that they were only here to 'civilize' us. Further, when it came to the teaching of our national history, there was wholesale distortion; indeed racism was used to deny us our own history. This, according to the imperialist occupiers, really only started after they had conquered and occupied our country.

In the classic fashion of imperialism, the Christian Church was used as the main instrument to wipe out our cultures and history. Again Cabral tells us that 'whatever may be the ideological or idealistic characteristic of cultural expression, culture is an essential element of the history of a people'[2] and to destroy it is essentially to destroy the historical roots of the people concerned. In this situation, the imperialists used the Christian Church to combat and destroy our cultures in the name of their god. The pulpit and the confession box were expertly used to propagate a bigoted imperialist culture among our people that was obsessed with prayer books, the bible and other religious fanaticism. From the pulpit the churchmen urged the Kenyan people to

1

accept their oppressed class position obediently, arguing that 'life and the development of society are the result of divine predestination.' 'Man proposes but God disposes' was the essence of their philosophy. In his novel, *Homecoming,* Ngugi wa Thiong'o tells us:

> But apart from the doctrine that poverty and the poor were blessed and would get their reward in heaven, the missionary preached the need to obey the powers that be. The saying 'render unto Caesar things that are Caesar's' was held up to the African churchgoers and schoolchildren. No matter how morally corrupt Caesar was, the African Christian was told to obey him. In this case Caesar was the colonial power. To tell the African that politics and political agitation was a dirty game and inconsistent with the Christian faith was a very easy step.[3]

The missionaries, fully backed by the secular forces of colonialism, burned and destroyed our material culture, calling it the handiwork of the devils; they adopted only those things of our spiritual and material cultures which they could use to facilitate colonial and racist indoctrination among our people. For instance, they condemned our national songs and dances as manifestations of Satan and, more telling, taught the Kenyan schoolchildren to detest them. I, for example, went to a school where we were severely punished if we happened to attend national festivals such as Muthuu, Muchungwa, and so on. It was considered a serious crime by white missionary teachers and their over-zealous local converts to sing these songs publicly. To be caught singing them meant outright expulsion from school. Therefore, I would like to make it very clear that the world 'Ngai' (literally, 'god') as it is used in these songs should not be interpreted literally, because the Ngai the people referred to during the heat of struggle was a material Ngai who symbolized their class unity and solidarity, their patriotism and heroism, and their correctness in the struggle. It was a fighting Ngai in the hearts of millions of oppressed Kenyans and not the Christian God who the imperialists and colonialists have created in their own image. The Ngai the people referred to was, is, anti-christianity, anti-colonialism and anti-imperialism.

We learn from Cabral that 'whatever may be the material aspects of [colonial] domination, it can be maintained only by the permanent, organized repression of the cultural life of the people concerned.'[4] In other words, the implantation of foreign domination can only succeed by physical liquidation of the spiritual and material cultures of the dominated nation and, in the process, by the elimination of the possibilities for cultural and political resistance by the nation. This was the main aim of the British colonialists in our country. But since they comprised only an insignificant minority, the colonialists had to rely on brutal coercion as well as on their economic power to maintain and build the system that suited their interests. In spite of being betrayed by Kenyan traitors, particularly Christian ones and the pro-colonial petty-bourgeois elite, the living core of most national cultures survived, amazingly in fact, having taken refuge in the villages and towns, in the forests, mountains and rivers of our country, and in the spirits of the broad masses of our people.

In resistance to the complete destruction of their cultures and history and to the imposition of imperialist culture, the Kenyan people, in the process, developed a new anti-colonial culture which found its expression in patriotic songs, poetry and dances such as Muthirigu[5] and in the anti-colonial movements such as Dini ya Musambwa, Dini ya Kaggia, Dini ya Roho, Ndonye ya Kati, Mumboism, etc.

Equally, the Kenya Independent School Movement formed the centre of a militant movement for cultural resistance. In fact, the leaders of the Independent School Movement were among the first to firmly express their hatred against the imposition of colonial culture in our country. They opposed and sabotaged its spread by leading militant demonstrations against it and propagating ideas of national patriotism amongst their students, thus frustrating and retarding the imperialist move to anglicize Kenyan culture. In this respect, these schools became a focal point of the anti-colonial cultural movement, and from their benches came not only simple teachers of the ABC but also patriotic and ardent fighters for the sacred cause of the liberation of our country. All in all, it was only when the Mau Mau Movement, led by the workers and peasants, stepped on to the stage of history that the anticolonial cultural movement became a powerful force capable of opposing and struggling against the spread of colonial culture. The Mau Mau songs, which were composed by the workers and peasants in the heat of resistance, marked the high point of Kenyans' anti-colonial cultural expression.

Besides being an expression of anti-colonial culture, these songs constitute an important pool of information, a kind of archive, on the Mau Mau Movement, which enables us to probe deeper into Mau Mau history and really understand its political objectives and methods. For us today these songs are an echo, a record, of our people's determination to liberate their country from foreign domination.

Specifically the songs eulogize the heroism of the Mau Mau guerrillas and sing the praises of those who distinguished themselves in destroying the enemy forces, and those others who made the ultimate sacrifice by hurling themselves into the cannon fire rather than fall into the hands of the imperialist hordes. They speak of mountains, valleys, forests, rivers and plains; of villages, towns and streets which were drenched in the blood of those gallant patriots who courageously laid down their lives for the liberation of their country. For instance, at the great Battle of Tumutumu Hill where the enemy forces met a total defeat, the song tells us:

> Burunji gave his own life
> To save the lives of his comrades,
> He lit the fuse and threw a grenade
> And their [enemy's] machine guns went dead
> Such a great victory for our guerrilla army.

3

These songs speak of thousands of Kenyans who sprinkled the battlefields with their blood. They sing of the great engagements which were fought and won by the Mau Mau guerrillas against the British forces and their local mercenaries. At the Battle of Timau we learn how successfully the Mau Mau guerrillas overran the enemy's air-base. The song goes:

> Who was in Timau when we attacked
> The airfield at Thundani's?
> Thebeni fired the first shot
> He fed the enemy with bullets.
>
> There was great rejoicing back
> At the coffee estate
> Because of our heroic deeds
> Under our leader's guidance.

After wiping out the enemy forces at the Battle of Naivasha,[6] a song was composed to immortalize our people's heroism:

> We rejoice and sing
> When we remember the Battle of Naivasha
> Thousands of words would not suffice
> To express our happiness;
> Thousands of songs would not suffice
> To praise our Mau Mau army
> We can only leap for joy
> And shout over and over again.

Similarly, to commemorate the Lukenya victory, a song was composed:

> When we arrived our fighters lay down;
> We opened fire and killed two guards.
>
> After fighting and releasing the prisoners,
> We prayed to Ngai in us
> So that he might assist us to return safely.
>
> All Black people of Nairobi were happy
> Congratulating us for our brave deeds.

The songs also speak of specific Mau Mau heroes. Among these heroes, the Mau Mau Generals hold a prominent place. Listen to the following examples from three different songs:

> The braves we sent
> To the Ndakaini Battle
> Were Kimathi and Kimemia
> They fought so courageously

And with such great dedication
That all the guerrillas
Were filled with joy.

The greatest patriots of Kenya today
Are Kimathi and Mathenge
Matenjagwo and Mbaria.

General Ihura, you are a great patriot
Get rid of the British
So that we have peace in the country.

Kimathi's unflinching leadership during the War and his fiercely militant political stance against the 'British/Christian/Taitai' alliance are well documented in many songs. In them he is recognized as the true leader of the Kenyan masses as well as the symbol of the country's heroism. One of the people's songs tells us:

Those with hearts of steel
Were made so by Kimathi
He recruited Kago
And then sent him to Nyandarwa
To fight for our liberation.

When the Kenyan masses were in distress and brutally oppressed, when thousands of them were sent to concentration camps and prisons to be tortured, when others were burned alive, raped and emasculated, they were not cowed because they confidently believed that, come what may, Kimathi would come to their rescue with the banner of freedom. This was a testimony to the potency of Mau Mau propaganda. A song entitled 'Kimathi Save Us From Slavery' reflects this:

Go quickly Kimathi
And save us from this slavery
Kenya is filled with bitter tears
Struggling for liberation.

Listen also to the following lines:

If I am called by Kimathi
I will go
He is our leader,
He is our liberator,
Let us embrace him.

Kimathi will identify
Those who have been oppressing us

> And the British will be driven out
> Together with their African puppets.

For the masses of Kenya and the guerrillas in the forest, Kimathi symbolized a new patriotism against foreign rule, he represented the birth of a new Kenya. He was the great inspirer in the heat of struggle. Even to this day, despite concerted attempts by anti-Mau Mau intellectuals,[7] the ex-Home Guards and other unpatriotic elements to brand Kimathi as a 'terrorist' and a 'brutal murderer', he still remains one of the most popular leaders and patriots in Kenya's history. To the majority of Kenyans Kimathi is the symbol of principled resistance to oppression. Other guerrilla leaders are also mentioned glowingly in several songs. Among them Generals Kago, Kariba, Ihura and Matenjagwo – all of them outstanding strategists. For instance, General Kariba heroically led the Mau Mau forces at the renowned Battle of Kaaruthi Valley which lasted for four days before the enemy forces were dispersed in humiliating defeat, thus:

> Most of the enemy soldiers
> Ran heading for Kiamacimbi
> They were using radio desperately
> Calling Nanyuki for reinforcements.

According to the song the enemy soldiers captured at the battle were executed on General Kariba's orders. He told his men:

> Concentrate on white soldiers first
> Leave the black puppets for the time being
> We will deal with them later.

For these Generals, victory meant national independence and the return of our stolen land. It is for that they gave their lives. Never did they entertain the idea of compromising with or surrendering to the enemy. All of them fell heroically in the field of battle. From one of the songs we learn that before his death at the great battle of Ndakaini, 'Gitau Matenjagwo put a handful of soil in his mouth and with his clenched fist held skyward, said, "I am dying as an African hero."'

During the Mau Mau war of national liberation our women did not flinch, they threw themselves into the struggle with great zeal and matchless heroism. In most cases it was the women who bravely rescued the Mau Mau forces from encirclement and annihilation. Women such as Kongania who, during the Battle of Tumutumu Hill, saved a large number of guerrillas from a terrible defeat. One of the people's songs goes:

> However, victory was with us
> Because Kongania, our woman contact,
> Brought us an important message

And thus saved a thousand lives.

It becomes clear that women shouldered a heavy burden in the war. They carried out every task assigned them in spite of the great risks involved. Thousands of them trudged day and night on hazardous routes and braved the enemy's wrath in order to supply the Mau Mau forces with food, medicine, ammunition and information. Others, with arms in their hands, joined the guerrilla army in the forest. Their heroism and patriotism, their iron determination and supreme self-sacrifice were obviously great contributions to the development of the Movement.

Finally, and most important, the songs speak out bitterly against those Kenyans, particularly the Home Guards, who betrayed the Movement to the British imperialists. In almost every song, it is made clear that the principal enemy of the Kenyan people was the British colonialists; and all those Kenyans who sided with them and helped them to oppress and kill the people were declared traitors. And war was declared on them, just as it was against the foreign occupiers. Listen to the following verses:

> You who sell us out are our great enemies
> Look around you and look at the British
> And also look at yourselves.
> The British are foreigners,
> And they will surely go back to their country
> Where will you, traitors to your country,
> Run to?

> And you traitors
> Who have joined forces with the enemy
> You will never be anything
> But the whiteman's slaves
> And when we win the war
> You will suffer for your betrayal.

Further, the songs make it very plain to the Kenyan mercenaries who were serving the British armed forces that, in helping the British to kill their compatriots, they were committing an act of treason against their nation and would be treated accordingly:

> We must continuously increase
> Our militant vigilance
> And intensify our battle
> Against these mercenaries and traitors
> Wiping them out one by one mercilessly.[8]

In the same vein the colonial puppet chiefs were attacked:

7

> Don't think you are a patriot,
> When you join the enemy forces,
> Remember that to betray your people
> Is an act of treason.
>
> Remember Nderi and Waruhiu
> Mbotela and Ofafa
> After they sold the country for money
> Where are they now?

The songs make it very clear to these traitors and murderers that, despite their treason, the Kenyan people would continue fighting until victory:

> We shall never, never give up
> Without land on which to grow food
> And without our own true freedom
> In our country of Kenya!

After highjacking our national independence in 1963, the remnants of these traitors, with full support of the ruling compradors, began to preach 'peace and brotherhood' — always invoking such slogans as 'enough blood has been shed', 'we all fought for independence', 'Let us forget the past', etc — in their attempt to make us forget the blood debts they owe. Since some of these individuals are now in positions of power and wealth, they have made it their main job to silence mercilessly any Kenyan patriot who speaks or writes about this heroic struggle. But if the past is any guide these efforts will be in vain. Two stanzas from the people's songs explain:

> You Home Guards must know
> We shall never forget that
> You had us put in prisons
> And treacherously revealed
> The secrets of the Africans.
>
> There can never be compromise with the traitors
> And no mercy towards them,
> For the blood of hundreds of our martyrs
> Cannot be forgotten
> And is crying for vengeance.[9]

8

References

1. Amilcar Cabral, *Return to the Source*, p.24.
2. *Ibid.*
3. Ngugi wa Thiong'o, *Homecoming*, p.33.
4. Amilcar Cabral, *op. cit.*, p.39.
5. Muthirigu was a powerful anti-colonial dance. It was banned by the British in January 1930, but continued to circulate underground as an echo of our people's resistance.
6. Unfortunately our contacts were not able to recollect the complete song of the Battle of Naivasha. We have recorded only three stanzas from it.
7. It would be fair to regard the following as leading anti-Mau Mau intellectuals: Dr. W.R. Ochieng, Senior Lecturer, Department of History, Kenyatta University College; Dr. B.E. Kiprorir, Director of Institute of African Studies, University of Nairobi; Professor B.A. Ogot, former Head, Department of History, University of Nairobi. See both Ochieng's and Kipkorir's articles in *Kenya Historical Review*, Vol.4., No.I, 1976, Nairobi, pp.138-43. For Professor Ogot see his works on the subject: 'Kenya Under the British, 1895 to 1963' in B.A. Ogot (ed.), *Zamani;* 'Revolt of the Elders', in B.A. Ogot (ed.), *Hadithi 4: Politics and Nationalism in Colonial Kenya,* 1972; and 'Politics, Culture and Music in Central Kenya: A Study of Mau Mau Hymns: 1951-1956', a paper presented to the Historical Association of Kenya in 1976. Dr. Atieno-Odhiambo, Senior Lecturer, Department of History, University of Nairobi, has also taken the same line in his recent article, 'Who were the Mau Mau?' in *African Perspectives*, No.2., Feb-March 1978. I have attacked this anti-Mau Mau line in my paper, 'The Peak of African Political Organization in Colonial Kenya', *Kenya Historical Review*, Vol.5, No.2, 1977.
8. The second stanza from the song of the Battle of Naivasha.
9. The third stanza of the song of the Battle of Naivasha.

PART 1
Mobilization Songs

I should like to remind those leaders who now condemn
Mau Mau and tell us to forget our past struggles and
suffering, that their present positions of power . . . would
not have been realized except for our sacrifices. I would
also warn them that we did not make these sacrifices just
to have Africans step into the shoes of our former
European masters.

The Urban Guerilla

I, for one, fail to understand why we should so easily forget
the great suffering endured by our people in the struggle for
land and freedom.

Man in the Middle

But I started thinking . . . Kimeria, who made his fortune
as a Home Guard transporting bodies of Mau Mau killed by
the British was still prospering . . .

Ngugi wa Thiong'o
Petals of Blood

The Message of the Workers

Chege's[1] message to the workers
Was given to Kubai
To preach to the masses.

Chorus
All over the world
Black people are suffering
And they ask: 'When will Chege return
So that we get our freedom?'

Before Mugo wa Kibiru[2] died,
He told us:
'When the railways have reached
Every corner of our country
The white people will go home.'

The workers will be happy
When we seize our freedom
Because they are the pillars of the country.

And Kaggia with Achieng will rejoice
Since they are the true patriots of the Kenyan masses.

The Song of Waiyaki [3]

I love being told the history of this land
When Waiyaki used to live on this our land
And how he so liked to see African people's progress
And I wish he were still amongst us today.

I would rejoice if he had shown us the tactics
That he used to agitate for our freedom

1. Refers to Chege wa Kibachia, the famous leader of the Kenyan trade union movement who was arrested and detained by the regime of the foreign occupiers from 1947 to 1957.
2. Mugo wa Kibiru was a patriotic prophet.
3. Waiyaki led the patriotic forces against the British invaders at the Battle of Dagoretti in 1890-92. First, he successfully destroyed the invading forces and burnt down their fortified depot. Later, after the foreign invaders had brought in reinforcements, Waiyaki was captured and taken to Kibwezi where he was brutally murdered. He was among the first Kenyan martyrs.

Or if I could just know his wisdom for struggle
To make us all realize that he was a true patriot.

We Kenyans must struggle even harder
So that we can get back our land,
The land taken from us by the British
Because they never came to this country with any land.

This struggle is the only way to inherit
A portion of Kenyan land
That was robbed from us long time ago,
When the British invaders deceived our elders.

All those who are being corrupted with bribes
They should know that we shall never abandon our land
Because it has been ours since Ndemi and Mathathi.[4]
They should know that
The children will continue the struggle.

The Curse of Waiyaki

Our people of Kenya,
It is good to work hard
So that our birthright is not stolen by the British.

Chorus
This is our land,
We the African people
Ngai blessed it for us
And he said we must never abandon it.

Our people! the foolish or the wise,
Who cannot see the wrongs
That the whites are heaping upon us
On top of all that exploitation
That we are going through.

---

4. The famous Gikuyu generation-sets.
5. Refers to Kenya Teachers College which was destroyed by the British forces during the Mau Mau war of national liberation. Literally 'thingira' means a man's special hut.

Chege wa Kibiru prophesied
That when the *Thingira* at Wairera[5]
Will be built and ready
We would surely get back our freedom.

And you our people who are in jails
And you who have been arrested
Because of your patriotism
Stop your tears and sorrows
For we will surely win the struggle.

Our people! Waiyaki died
And he left us a serious curse:
We should never sell out our land.
And yet we are now giving it away!

The whites are foreigners
They will one day leave this our country
Where will you traitors run to
When the Kenyan masses gather in victory?

May Imperialism Perish Forever

I love reading about Chege[6]
About the time when he lived here on earth
I wish I was present
When he used to prophesy that
The colonialists would invade our country
And that they would be driven right out again.

I shall be delighted when I see
The colonialists going back to their own country
So that our children will have their freedom
And live in peace in our own country,
The same way their children live in their country.
Imperialists, may you vanish and perish forever!

Nature gave us this land
And provided us with rich black soils
Black like the colour of our skins.

6. Chege wa Kibiru was a patriot and a prophet.

15

He also provided us
With many beautiful streams and great rivers
But now the colonialists have seized
All of them from us.

Those who have ears, listen:
Hardships and suffering
Were experienced by our people in Olenguruone.[7]
They endured heavy rains and severe cold,
But they refused to submit to the enemy's demands,
They firmly declared:
'We shall never surrender our land
To the foreign occupiers!'

Our people, let us welcome our heroes home
With patriotic love.
Let us share with them land and livestock
We have snatched from the enemy.

Countrymen!
Our enemy has oppressed us,
He has stolen our land
And our livestock
But we shall never surrender,
We shall fight with heroism
Until we drive him out of the country.

Struggle For Our Land

I am amazed,
My heart is truly amazed,
Because of the things
That Chege prophesied would come to be.

Chorus
Struggle for our land!
Struggle for our land!

7. On October 29, 1949, 11,000 Gikuyu peasants were forcibly evicted from their land
   in Olenguruone to make room for the white settlers. Because the peasants put up a
   bitter resistance against the eviction, the majority of them were arrested and detained
   at Yatta.

Because the land was ours
But was taken from us.

Chege prophesied before he died:
'Conflict and hatred will increase
And friendships will diminish.'

Chege will be reborn in us
And when he comes back
You'll get your freedom.

And when he returns
You'll be unable to recognize him
Because of those who are abusing his memory
And throwing insults upon his name.

Don't mind being hated and being abused
Because those who are abusing his memory
Have no goats and no land,
They have no cows, they are traitors.
They are just telling lies about him
Because they hear colonialists doing it,
Aping colonialists but ignorant of the reason why!

Wherever a Black man is now dwelling
There is conflict and struggle.
Even if you remain sycophantic,
You are still a Black man!

Now Chege has come back
And still you don't know it
Those who abused his memory
Look for a place to hide.

Why Sell Your Land?

This land belonged to Gikuyu
Ngai created and gave it to his chosen ones,
Gikuyu and Mumbi[8] to live there.

---

8. Gikuyu and Mumbi are the original parents of the Gikuyu nationality.

The seer Mugo wa Kibiru said:
'Pink and white butterflies
Will come from the East
And later will vanish.'

And Mugo was given a walking-stick for leadership
Like the one which was given to Musa in Misri
To lead the Children of Gikuyu.

Bless him to watch carefully over your children.
The stone which the Builders refused
Is the same stone they later used.

Agikuyu! why throw away your proverbs
When you know them?
You said: 'Unity is strength',
And again, 'The lazy ones don't have cows'.

Our people! why sell your land,
Because of your stomachs?
Knowing very well that the stomach
Will never be satisfied
While your land is everlasting.

When the British Came

When the British came here from Europe
They told us they only brought us learning
And we received them with suspicion.
Wuui, iiya,[9] they only came to oppress us!

Those who hate their fellow Africans
And claim they love the British,
They will be punished the day
We regain our freedom.

Whenever African people gather
There are some traitors
Who rush information to the oppressor
Very much like the Judas of old.

9. Wuui, iiya, or uui, iiyai, or wui, wui, are all cries of suffering.

18

Our people! no matter how much they torture you
Have no fear in your hearts.
There is an old proverb which says:
'Ngai helps those who help themselves.'

And you who fawn on the British oppressors,
When they return to their homes in Europe
You will have to kneel before us, crying:
Wuui, we did not know this would come to us.

The day the foreigners return to Europe
We shall all turn to those who sold us to them,
We shall tell them: 'We reject you!
Didn't you denounce and betray us?'

Those people who betray us
May they be cursed with their own traitorous deeds,
And if it is because of the money they are given,
May the money turn against them.

Tell the Elders to Keep Quiet

Dear parents and friends,
We pray you listen to us
Speaking out openly with malice to none.

Chorus
Tell the elders to keep quiet
They let our land be taken.
Tell the young to rise up in arms
So that this land may be returned to us.

When the imperialists came with wiles
They told us they had come to bring us education
But they had come to eat us alive.

The time has now come
For us to open our ears and eyes,
And even our hearts we should open.

Our whole country is in darkness
And the squatters increase daily
And when the youth want to rise up

19

They are cautioned that the time is not ripe!

The Need for Spears Is Gone

Problems have never solved themselves
Difficulties are there to be surmounted
The wise and even the foolish:
Who has not got ears!
Who has not heard the anguish of our children!

Now that there are no schools for Africans' children
The British oppressor does not mind
And neither does the Indian merchant lose his sleep
Worrying over what will benefit our children tomorrow.

This is the time to struggle:
Kenyans come forward
And build many revolutionary schools all over Kenya[9a]
We have suffered enough.

The days of relying solely on spears are gone.
Now it is time to add the power of the pen to the spear
Because our enemies today
Also add the power of their pens to their arms.

And you, our parents, give us pens
So that when the enemy attacks us
We shall come forward and assist our patriots —
For the youth must be ready
To take the place of the aged.

Let us all be ready to fight for our land
And let the children sharpen their minds
And those amongst us who have turned traitor
May the curse of the children befall them!

Father, I Now Demand Education

If it were the time of Ndemi and Mathathi
Father, I would demand a feast of bulls

9a. The Kenyan people organized their own schools to combat imperialist education; they later became recruitment bases for the armed struggle.

And after, I would demand of you a spear and a shield,
But now, father, all I demand of you is education.

Now there are no bulls anymore
And the goats decrease daily
So I cannot ask you for any feast
But now, father, I ask you for education.

My mother has often told you
And I have also declared to you
That I will never demand any feast
Father, I want only education.

For a present-day hero
His warrior's victory dance is education!
Is it not education that has made Mathu[10] a hero?
How else shall I be able to dance proudly the victory dance?

Father, all of the Kenyan patriots have united
To defend our land against the British oppressors,
Why have you not thought of joining them?

We Are Building Our Own School

Go to Githunguri to see the school of Kenyan people
It is in a four-storey building.

The builders are Kenyan
The chief overseer is a Kenyan
The building committee is Kenyan
And the money has been contributed by Kenyans.

The Seer predicted that
The base of the liberation of Kenya
Would be at Githunguri.

---

10. The nomination of Mathu to the Legislative Council in 1944 was first seen as a
    victory over British colonialism by our people. But later, after his failure to represent
    the interests of the Kenyan masses inside and outside the Legislative Council, he
    was denounced by the people. In fact, Mathu was one of the Kenyans who were
    marked down for elimination by the Mau Mau guerrillas because of their
    collaboration with the enemy.

21

We must build this centre for our education,
Otherwise the British will humiliate us forever.

Mwene-Nyaga unite us together
So that we can together shoulder
All the problems facing us Kenyans!

Thai, thai Ngai! Thai, thai Ngai![11]
Our unity and solidarity
Should be firm as a rock!

Study Hard, Children

Ngai of the Black people
Help the children
As they ask for rain;
Ngai hear the prayers of the people
And let the rains fall.

And you boys and girls, study hard!
In the struggle for our land.
As for those who sell our land
To the foreign invaders
You will put your anguished heads together
And plot their downfall.

When we are struggling for freedom,
Often being imprisoned and whipped for nothing,
We the masses of the country should never
Allow ourselves to be corrupted by whites with money.

If you allow yourselves to be corrupted
And you become an agent,
Spilling the blood of the people,
Rejecting KAU's political programme,
You will be treated just like Judas.

If you struggle in unity
We shall get our freedom.

11. Literally, Thaai or Thai means 'peace'; Thaai Ngai Thai means 'in peace we pray, O
    God; and Thaai, Thathaiya Ngai Thai means 'O God, hear our prayers for peace.'

Don't Be Sad, Our Children

Don't be sad, Father
Don't be sad, Mother
Don't be sad
Don't be sad.
We will get the land back
Which was stolen from you by the whites.

Don't be sad, my brothers.
We will get the land back
Which was stolen from you by the whites.
Don't be sad, my brothers.

Don't be sad, our children.
We will get the land back
Which was stolen by the whites,
So don't be sad.

Don't be sad, our compatriots.
We will get the land back
Which was stolen by the whites.
So don't be sad.

Our land will be returned
Which was stolen by the whites.
So don't be sad
We will get our land back.

Parents Help the Children

We salute you, beloved parents,
For this is a fitting day
For us to put our thoughts together.

Chorus
*Wui, Wui, parents help your children
In the struggle for freedom.*

Parents help the children
In the struggle for freedom;
Give them advice through actions
Our liberation is near.

Don't take it that what you contribute
Is like a gift thrown away.
You will be repaid by the nation
A thousand times.

What is in your pocket
Can only speak through your actions
Don't deny yourself the gratitude
Of the children and the whole nation.

If you give freely
You will be freely given by the nation.
If you become a good student
You will become a good teacher.

You used to be impatient for action!
Yes, only hard work and commitment
Can bring about our liberation.

Inheritance of Gikuyu

Ngai created Gikuyu and Mumbi
And he gave them land for their children
Which has now been stolen by foreigners.

Chorus
Wuui, children were wailing
Because of being oppressed.
Wuui, let us weep for Gikuyu and Mumbi,
Are we all going to perish?

He who only thinks of his own personal gains
Must remember that Gikuyu once said that
Such a person will never benefit the people.

Let the hypocrites of the land remember that
A time will come
When they will be like Judas!

Time has now come
To fight the foreign oppressors.
The oath was given to make people think.

Parents, help to educate the children
Until all of them become wise,
So that they may help you
In the fight for our land.

I Will Search My Heart

Now search you all your hearts
And pray to Ngai.
Why do you reject your roots
In Gikuyu and Mumbi
To follow a white man, this big ogre!

Chorus
I now ask in my heart
Shall I ever see with my own eyes
The liberation of Kenya.

Know that roots in our past are important!
If you don't inherit your past,
You will inherit oppression,
You will inherit death and poverty
And this is the beginning of ignorance.

The British have plotted against you,
You Mumbi and Gikuyu
But you must remain steadfast like Waiyaki.
Even when they detained and killed him,
Waiyaki never rejected his roots.

How dare you cultivate a *shamba*[12]
And make friends with wild animals!
You'll one day cry and even make me cry
When you have nothing to harvest.

12. A Swahili word meaning 'plot of land'.

25

Holder of the Plough

If the ploughman were to keep on
Looking back over his shoulder
The ploughshare would jump over sections
Leaving patches uncultivated.

Chorus
Mwene-Nyaga abhors those with two hearts
He hates to be given half hearts
He is jealous
And He never likes to be given pieces.
Give him all your heart
And He will be happy.

Ngai is a hero of war.
He is a witness to what He told his people:
'It is not good to just talk
Without putting words into practice.'

Let your rejoicing be turned into mourning
And your laughter become sorrow.
Aware that you are being oppressed,
Encourage the braves of the nation
To fight for our land.

You barren ones, traitors of the land,
Take care!
Because the curse is upon you
For selling out the country
And the freedom of Black people!

And the curse which is upon you
Is the curse put on you by Mugo wa Kibiru
When he said: 'In the country of the Black people,
There will be born people with bells in their ears!'[13]

13. That is, there will be individuals born who would betray their own people to
foreigners.

The Traitors To Our Cause

Ngai of Mumbi and Gikuyu
Does not shut his ears
To our cries and anguish
Because our land was taken.

Ngai of Mount Kenya
Who gave us this land,
Hear our cries.
Take back the whites to their country
They left their land
To come to rob and oppress us.

And you traitors of our cause
Remember you too have children!
You went to the side of the enemy.
When the enemy returns to his country
You will pay for your treachery.

They deceived and told us to pray
That if we closed our eyes in prayer we would get strength
But it is our land which was taken instead.
Where will our children go now?
Fight that we get our land back!

The General Cry in Gikuyuland

Chege bequeathed leadership
To Mwangi and Irungu generations
Never throw away this elder son's birthright
In the House of Mumbi.

Chorus
There is general crying in Gikuyuland
Of those whose lands were stolen
Asking themselves: 'When will Chege return
So we can get back our land?'

Gikuyu prays to Ngai
Standing under the sacred fig tree
And holding for sacrifice a ram without blemish.

Gikuyu had fertile earth, full of milk and honey,
Full of yams and bananas,
Goats and cattle.

Colonial laws were brought into Gikuyuland,
Laws that took from us all our wealth:
Goats, cattle and land.

After Gikuyu fought against the Germans,
Using shields and spears and sharp arrows,
He did not receive any rewards.

Now we beseech you Creator of earth
Hear our prayers
Grant us all we are asking for,

Foreigner in this homestead
Pack your bags and go
For the owner of the house has arrived!
Put down decorations that
Do not belong to you!
Did you think I was going to perish,
Never to come back?

Never Sell Out the Country

Ngai gave us this country a long time ago
When he was dividing up the earth among all nations.
And he said we should never give it up,
But we were robbed of it
By those colonial hordes that invaded our country.
Ngai, we shall get back our land.

Ngai remembers his children
Those he left here in Kenya
And he is aware of their sufferings
He now has sent his cadres
That he has selected from amongst us
To lead the struggle for freedom.

He has sent light to his children
To guide them here in Kenya.
Before they did not have it

And that is why they were robbed of their land.
Now they have seen his light
And they are fearlessly demanding
The return of their land.

All the nationalities in Kenya
Should know that KAU's guidelines
Have become our sword of justice
Which will destroy the power of our enemy.

Before Waiyaki died, he said:
'Never sell out or betray our land
Because land is the source of all wealth.'
Why are you now selling it,
Have you forgotten the curse of Waiyaki?

The Betrayer

Long ago the British came upon us
With weapons of war
And they successfully fought us
And drove us out and took our land.
Go away, go away, you whites,
The time is soon coming
When you will be crying for mercy.

There is a great wailing
In the land of the African people
Because of land hunger.
The wise and even the foolish,
Who among you does not see
The overcrowding in our land?

You whites are like beasts in sheep's clothing
You pretended you came to lead us into the light
But instead you stole our land.
Go away, go away, you whites,
The years that are past
Have been more than enough for us!

You divided us into police and common people
So that if the common people put up a resistance
They are viciously punished by their traitorous brothers

And yet the Black policeman is himself oppressed.
Go away, go away, you whites,
The years that are past
Have been more than enough for us!

You who betray the people,
I ask myself what will happen to you
When the whites have gone back to their own land.
Go away, go away, you whites,
The years that are past
Have been more than enough for us!

The Flag Belongs to the Kenyans

African people, *thaai, thaai!*
Thai Thathaiya Ngai, thaai, thaai!

We are agitating for our land, *thaai, thaai!*
Left to us by Iregi,[14] *thaai, thaai!*

Walk in dignity, *thaai, thaai!*
This country is ours, *thaai, thaai!*

Now lift up your eyes, *thaai, thaai!*
To see us being sold for money by the traitors, *thaai, thaai!*

Our centre will be seen, *thaai, thaai!*
Up there at Githunguri, *thaai, thaai!*

We shall be grazing our livestock, *thaai, thaai!*
On the land of the African people, *thaai, thaai!*

We reject secret deals, *thaai, thaai!*
Everyone must come openly to the masses, *thaai, thaai!*

Don't take bribes, *thaai, thaai!*
To sell out your country, *thaai, thaai!*

14. Iregi was a rebellious generation-set that said 'No' to internal oppression and over-
threw the tyrannical rule of the Kings. It was the first generation to celebrate
Ituika (revolution) in Gikuyuland.

A person who wants to be cursed, *thaai, thaai!*
Let him accept bribes, *thaai, thaai!*

Let us demand back our land in unity, *thaai, thaai!*
Because it is our birthright, *thaai, thaai!*

The flag belongs to the Kenyans, *thaai, thaai!*
Thaai, thathaiya Ngai, thaai, thaai!

Draughts Players

You draughts players are always in hotels,
You move the pieces for whom?
The British oppressors are waiting to do their devilish work!
Whom will you blame when you become poor?

Young man, when the sun rises in the morning
You are already anxious for daylight to come
So you may run to the market!
And after you drink a bottle of beer and tea in hotels,
How will playing draughts benefit you?

If a young man forgets the draughts
He remains healthy for many days.
Run to your *shamba* and get your blessing!
If you keep at work you'll get rich.

You draughts-player clan
Run to KAU and get blessings to last you many years;
KAU is not in darkness but in the light
If you have faith come and let's unite!
Because *rwi komu rwi na kaigu wa nyina.* [15]

Struggle Brings Peace

After a season of danger and sufferings

15. A Gikuyu proverb, meaning literally 'the fate of the dry stick awaits the green stick, its brother'.

There follows a season of happiness.
And after a season of happiness
There follows a season of misery and calamities.
Pause, pause, and think hard.

If only you would search your hearts
And know that
He who serves others can also be served,
And a man in authority
Can be reduced to nothing if rejected,
You would pause, pause and think hard.

The proudest time is
When you are helping the masses!
Remember he who starts with plenty
Is not he who ends with plenty.
Pause, pause and think hard.

Or are you the one
About whom it has been said:
A fool is like a beehive
He can be hanged in any way,
Perhaps if you have been hanged that way,
You would realize the reason why.
Pause, pause and criticize yourself.

In your place there was once a potter,
Didn't you see her cooking in broken pots?
Know yourself because
Rwi itara no mitheko[16]
Pause, pause and think hard.

If you don't get to know these things
You will be rejected by the House of Mumbi!
When a piece of firewood is pushed into the fire
It fills the whole house with smoke.
Pause, pause and cleanse yourself of leprosy.

If water could make you clean
I would wash you clean so you may know
Patriotism is more important than wealth.
Pause, pause and give yourself
To the service of your country.

16. A Gikuyu metaphor meaning literally 'the firewood laughs at the embers.'

The Indomitability of Kang'ethe [17]

Who was present at Kang'ethe's home
On April the 13th
And witnessed the deed that was done
Yes, that was done by the enemies of our nation.

Chorus
I know nothing else but this:
I will always praise the people's heroes.
I know no other song but this:
To praise the national patriots.

Ngai of Black people does not sleep.
The wronged one does not
Always fall into the pit intended for him.
And he who hurls an object
Does not always know who will escape it.
Ngai of the Black people, help us.

There were fifteen Black policemen
And two white police officers
Armed with sticks.
The Black policemen had guns
They had come to make the nation suffer.

I witnessed great sorrow.
Children and women were crying:
'Oh, shall we all perish?'

But Kang'ethe told them courageously:
'Our people, don't you run away
We have not stolen or murdered
Let us rather die together!'

A wealthy Gikuyu tried to save himself
He told the police:
'I did not come for the tea,[18]
I came to fetch my dogs.'

17. Joseph Kang'ethe was one of the founders of the Kikuyu Central Association (KCA) in 1924. He served the Association as its President for more than 15 years. When the Association was banned by the colonial occupationists in 1940, Kang'ethe and other patriots were arrested and detained at Kapenguria. After Uhuru, because of his bitter opposition to the Kenyan ruling compradors, who, have turned the country into a backyard of imperialism, Kang'ethe was eliminated.
18. That is, 'I did not come to take the Mau Mau oath'.

This coward of wealth
Thought all were going to perish.
I beseech you, don't be afraid
Don't you realize that to be jailed
Is only a bridge toward liberation?

Forty people were arrested
The enemy was very happy about this
But you traitors should realize that
When the white colonialists leave our country
You will pay for your treachery with your lives.

The women who were left behind
And watched as the people were driven away,
Instead of falling into despair
They trilled the *Ngemi*[19] for courageous sons!

You traitors you sell our people
Don't you read the KAU guidelines
And hear what they say:
'Love your country as you love yourself.'

All those who were arrested
Not one of them was frightened at all
They firmly told their captors:
'Quick and hurry!
Take us wherever you want to!'

Luckily the enemy was not able
To arrest most of the cadres,
Ngai was on our side.

And all the parents
Now broke into joyful ululations
Then they said: 'All praises to Ngai!
And don't be afraid,
For the fighting Ngai is within us.'

19. Ngemi means 'ululations' in Gikuyu.

Saturday Night

On Saturday night
We received an important message:
That our leaders would be at Kaloleni.
But when we got there
They had not yet arrived.

After waiting for a while
We suddenly heard thunderous handclaps
And the trilling of voices
Were themselves like thunder.
The women's group said:
'Give five patriotic ululations
For our leaders have come!'

We were thirty-five thousand strong,
And in one single voice we firmly declared:
'We shall never give up the fight for our land
And freedom for our country!'

The Kaloleni Meeting

One day KAU leaders met at Kaloleni
And they decided to go into secret session
To plan for the recovery of our land.

Chorus
Call all the Kenyan masses
And let us now plan secretly
We are full of indignation
Because of our soil
Which has been taken from us
By the foreign occupiers.

Firstly they declared:
'We shall never cease to agitate
For the return of our stolen land!'
Secondly they emphatically said:
'We will continue with the struggle
Until we seize our freedom.'

We are overcrowded in our homes

And we no longer have good grazing grounds
And we no longer have good land for growing crops
But we are always forced
To dig useless trenches.[20]

Let each and everyone ask himself:
'Where do I stand in the struggle
Of the African people?'
For the time is soon coming
When, like the days of long ago,
Evil people will be burned
And wiped off the face of the earth.

Pray and fight hard all you,
Children of African people,
So that we can seize our freedom.
We shall rejoice, all of us African people,
When the land is returned to us.

You British oppressors make merry now,
For the day is coming when you will weep.
Because of all the evils you have done to us
And shall drive you out
And make you perish in the sea!

Our Delegation Was Sent to the U.N.O.

It was a day of fortune
When we sent our delegation.
It was the first time
We ever sent any delegation to the U.N.O.

Chorus
It was a beautiful day
When we sent our delegation.
It was the first time

20. Between 1948 and 1950 the Colonial Government of Kenya forced a soil conservation law on the Kenyan peasants. When the peasants resisted this evil law, the
colonial regime brought in the police. As a result, the peasant masses under James
Beauttah's leadership organized an anti-soil conservation movement in Murang'a
District.

We ever sent any delegation to the U.N.O.
To explain our situation to the world body,
It was in truth a beautiful day
The day they took the flight.

Now no African can sleep
Because of lack of adequate food.
We shall be happy
When we get our land back.

In great unity
The Kenyan people truly united
Let us now throw this colonial yoke off our backs
So we can find open fields in which to work and play.

We shall be very happy
When our oppressors are forced to agree
That we are the masters of this land.
Today they call us 'boys'
Because they pretend not to know who we are!

Our fertile land was taken from us
We were forced into desert land
And still they continue to treat us
As if an African has no blood in his veins.

Our delegates will tell us
To await them at the airport
It is not money they will bring to us
But something that will benefit us to eternity.

Wipe Out the Traitors

Our people, we sent a delegation to London
To fight for our stolen land.
So when you eat and drink happily
Remember that they are still in London.

Chorus
You who are present
Aren't you sad,
Aren't you full of tears,
Remembering that we were robbed of our land?

Greed will never be satisfied,
Why do you therefore have to sell
The Kenyan people for money,
When we are about
To get back our land
And regain our freedom?

You traitors who torture our people
You will pay with your lives
For your evil deeds,
Kenyans will decide your fate.

Our people are filled with indignation
Towards your treachery.
If you don't repent
And cease your treasonable activities
You will be wiped out.

Don't be corrupted by money,
Fight for the soil
That was left to us
By our forefathers.

Mugo wa Kibiru said:
'There will come an oppressor
And he will rob you of your country.'
And that is exactly what has happened.

I Will Repent Now

I have aimlessly wandered all over the country
I will now repent
I will repent without a shred of doubt,
So have mercy and forgive me.

Chorus
I will come back to you, our people,
So teach me,
Because of the love of the country
Have mercy and receive me.

I will give my reasons
I will now repent
I will abandon my double-dealing ways
I will truly repent.

From the days of Ndemi and Mathathi
The land has always been ours
All the trenches should be covered
Since Africans are suffering from digging them.

I ask Koinange wa Mbiyu:
'Whose children are forced
To pick up coffee-beans,
Aren't they our children?'

The coffee plantation overseer,
You are condemned by the whole country.
Come, repent before the people.

This Country is Ours

Kaggia tells us join KAU
And to follow its leaders so that
We can defeat the colonialists and their lackeys.

You British are foreigners
In this country of the African people.
Deep down in your hearts you know
That you will have to return to your homes.

You who have agreed to be
The running dogs of the British,
The African people condemn you forever.

Gikuyu was told by Murungu:
'Do you see all this land?
I want you and your children's children
To dwell on it forever.'[21]

Even if you oppress us

21. This refers to the myth of Gikuyu and his Ngai at the top of Mount Kirinyaga.

This country belongs to us
We were given it by Murungu
And we shall never abandon it.

Mwene-Nyaga in the millions of us
We will drive the foreigners out of the country
And we, the African people,
Will remain triumphant
Since this is our country.

Let Us Worship the National Heroes

Come, let us weep and fight together
It is really painful to see
Our land being taken by foreigners.

We had inherited enough land,
But see, we don't have enough land now.
The foreigners laugh in our faces
As they milk the wealth of our country.

The stupidity of people like Mbotela and Ofafa[22]
Is very dangerous to our cause;
It has made them sell the country
To the white oppressors.

Now let us worship the heroes of the country
They will fight for our land
Until we get all of it back.

Freedom Will Never Be Achieved by the Lazy

We made a great covenant with Gikuyu:
He said he would never desert us
And Murungu would never abandon us.

---

22. Mbotela and Ofafa were eliminated by the Mau Mau partisans for their treachery in 1952.

Chorus
Do you truly say
Truly say you'll never desert us,
Or will you look back regretfully?

If you sell the nation to enrich yourself
Know that the curse will be upon your house.
When Judas betrayed Jesus,
He ended up dying a rotten death.

Be sad and afterwards ask yourself:
What benefit do you really get
Happily eating and laughing
When others are crying?

Remember Nderi and Waruhiu,[23]
Mbotela and Ofafa,
After they sold the country for money,
Where are they now?

Know that the freedom we are fighting for
Will never be achieved by mere words,
It will be achieved through great toil!
And it will never be achieved by the lazy!

Who Has Eyes But Does Not See?

Who has eyes and cannot see?
It is he who cannot see for the nation.

Who is it that has ears and cannot hear?
It is he who cannot hear for the nation.

Who is it that travels, but never arrives?
It is he who cannot walk on behalf of the nation.

Wuui, Wuui, Africans shall we perish one by one?
Wuui, Wuui, shall we watch passively,
While we are being exterminated?

---

23. Nderi and Waruhiu were colonial chiefs. They were eliminated in 1952 by the
Mau Mau partisans for their treachery.

The Call

There is no success without a struggle
What are you waiting for?
Where are you when the struggle for land is on,
What are you waiting for?

Chorus
What are you waiting for
The moment has come,
What are you waiting for?

Have you not yet joined,
What are you waiting for?
Join our Mau Mau army,
What are you waiting for?

Even if you think you are rich,
What are you waiting for?
Land is truly our national wealth,
What are you waiting for?

What sort of man are you,
What are you waiting for?
Or are you one of the whites,
What are you waiting for?

And you, man of religion,
What are you waiting for?
Remember land is the source of national strength,
What are you waiting for?

Even if you think you are too important,
What are you waiting for?
Let us unite in struggle,
What are you waiting for?

Unity is strength,
What are you waiting for?
Mau Mau is the people's movement,
What are you waiting for?

We are struggling for our liberation,
What are you waiting for?
Don't you yourself like to be free,
What are you waiting for?

The Book of Gikuyu

The book of Gikuyu is holy
It helps me to be honest
It is my political guide
When I join the people's army.

The book is 'Mau Mau'
It shows me the way
To fight for the liberation of my country
And free it from British slavery.

The book will guide me
So that I persist to love
My country all my life.

If I accept its guidelines
I will never be called 'boy' again
I will get freedom through Mau Mau.

Listen, Come All of You

To our parents together with our friends
Those we were born with:
Listen, this country is in a great turmoil
Because our land was stolen.

Chorus
Listen, come!
Our land was stolen
But remember it will be returned.

Why did the whites
Come to our country?
They brought misery,
They stole our land and killed our livestock.
We are now beggars in our own country.

Don't be deceived with money,
Don't be tempted to sell our country to foreigners
The Movement demands nothing
But unity among our people
So that we can fight for our stolen land together.

And you traitors
Who have joined forces with the enemy
You will never be anything
But white men's slaves,
And when we win the war
You will suffer for your betrayal.

Firstly, you colonialists detained Waiyaki,
Secondly, you killed him,
Thirdly, you arrested and detained Chege.
All of this, we shall never forget.

The Mau Mau guidelines explain
That the Kenyan society
Has been divided into two opposing forces:
The people and their Mau Mau army on the one hand,
And the traitors of the land and British colonialism on the other.

The Nyeri Rally of 1952

The women's lorry was the first to start
It left Nairobi at eight in the morning
And it arrived in Nyeri at noon
Where the patriotic youth were waiting for us.

Chorus
We shall greatly rejoice
When we get our land back
And freedom for our country.

Women were sad and greatly worried
For they had not yet seen the leader.
When they saw him they were happy
And made thunderous ululations.

We became extremely concerned
After receiving bad news about our heroes
Who were being tortured in Murang'a.
They were saved by Ngai of our struggle.

Kimathi came with three battalions
Mathenge asked them to get organized
With Nyeri leaders in front

And women to follow with ululations.

We were really moved when the song
Castigating the lazy ones was sung.
Old men and women were extremely disturbed
Since it reminded them
How some had sold the land to the foreign invaders.

We saw many unbelievable things:
The agents of colonialism tried to woo
Our leaders on to their side.
But they did not succeed
They failed.

A colonialist with a camera
Stood in front of the masses
Ready to take their pictures.
The militant words of the leaders
Prevented this foreign spy
From collecting any useful information.

May This Soil Damn You Forever

Wake up all of you
From Ngong to Karimatura[24]
We have found the beast
We have been looking for.
Wake up quickly and let us face it.

When you hear a thunderous noise
You should know that it is not rain
Or thunder clouds.
It is the guerrillas heading toward Nyandarwa
To fight for our freedom.

Spear-bearing traitor
Hiding in the homestead
Should be kicked out
With his miserable stolen belongings.
The rightful owner of the homestead has returned

24. Refers to the Garba Tula Hill in Isiolo District.

Holding the freedom torch firmly in his hand.

Njiiri,[25] you and your Home Guard traitors
You have sold this country for money
You have also sold our Kimathi for money
Where will you go when we seize our freedom?
May this soil damn you forever.

You British oppressors,
You think your luck will hold forever
Because you have your own land in Europe
And now you want to take Kenya from us.
The day we seize our freedom
You will face the wrath of Kenyans.

May the seller of the country
Breaks his limbs
And his backbone rot in shame.

We Shall Never Compromise

It was at one in the afternoon
When the KAU leaders were all arrested.

Chorus
The settlers mocked them, saying:
You have defended the Africans
Now defend yourselves.
If you can win,
We will believe you.

When KAU leaders got inside the plane
We received a secret message
That they had arrived in N.F.D.[26] safely.

The white settlers were laughing at us
And insulting us as well.

25. Njiiri was a colonial chief. Under the protection of the British forces, Njiiri and
     his clique of traitors murdered many innocent Kenyans in Murang'a District during
     the struggle.
26. The colonial occupiers used to refer to the northern region of our country as the
     Northern Frontier District.

They told us that our leaders will never return.

When Pritt received the news in London
He felt strong sympathy
Seeing the Kenyans in trouble.

We were much embarrassed at the court
To learn that those who witnessed against us
Were our own brothers and sisters.

Pritt asked a traitorous girl, Peninah Wanjiku:
'Are you sure Jomo was there
When the oath was administered?'
And she was unable to answer the question.

You Home Guards must know
We shall never forget that
You had us put in prisons
And treacherously revealed the secrets of the Africans.

When the Emergency is ended
We will return home
And many Home Guards will commit suicide.

Let Us Die If Need Be

Our people, during our forefathers' days
This country was defended by the army
With people armed with weapons of war,
Why do you want to shame our forefathers now?

Those who are indifferent
Because we are demanding our land
And freedom for our country,
Haven't they yet realized
Why we took the oath?

We took the oath
In order to fight for our land
And freedom for African people.
Truly slavery is evil
And you are perpetuating it.

Those who live on bribery
Where will they run to,
When we seize our freedom?
You will kneel down before us and weep!

Those who are not in the Movement
Come quickly and join
So that we shoulder this sacred task together
As the saying goes: 'Unity is strength'.

Let us try to share
This great work of the masses
And show our commitment for sure,
For the future of this country
Depends on you and me.
Let us die if need be
For our children's future!

Our enemy is the British colonialists
They are powerful and vicious
They torture and murder our patriots,
But with faith and commitment
We will surely triumph.

Freedom! Freedom! Freedom!

We salute you all, parents and friends,
And we thank Ngai for making it possible
For us to gather here.

Chorus
Freedom! Freedom! Freedom!
Freedom for this country of Kenya,
A land of happiness
With rich soil and beautiful forests.
Kenya is an African people's country.

Hail, hail to the national patriots
Great heroes of our country.
The country and her children
Depend on your courageous leadership
Fight hard for the future of the children.

Let us unite together our compatriots
And forget tribalism and disunity
The foolish or the clever, the rich or the poor:
We should all realize
That our great aim is *Freedom!*

You, my father and my mother,
And even you my friend,
Lift your eyes and ask yourselves:
'Where is our country heading to?'

Children are the future of the country,
They are inherited from Ngai.
This country is ours
And it is our birthright.
Ngai, protect our inheritance.

We are not afraid of detention
Or of being locked in prisons
Or of being deported to remote islands
Because we shall never cease
To struggle and fight for liberation
Until our country is free!

You traitors who love foreign things and luxuries
Remember that these things cannot be equal to our country,
And they will never satisfy your stomachs.
This country is ours,
Our own inheritance from Ngai,
It is ours for ever and ever.

PART 2
Detention Songs

I don't know what the future has in store for me. I can only hope that with Kenya's independence my suffering of the past ten years will somehow be rewarded . . . Only I pray that after independence our children will not be forced to fight again.

The Hardcore

I am filled with great regret on realization of the fact that the forest fighters' survivors, the widows and orphans of those who volunteered to sacrifice their lives in order to liberate the Kenya nation from colonial rule, have no place to enjoy the fruits of their fallen parents' and husbands' labour.

Mau Mau From Within

As I sold sheepskins to Watalii I asked myself, how could a whole community be taken in by a few greedy stomachs — greedy because they had eaten more than their fair share of that which was bought by the blood of the people.

Ngugi wa Thiong'o
Petals of Blood

The Olenguruone Struggle

The name of the Black people's Ngai
Is true and holy and consecrated.
That is why the patriarch forbade
Its being mouthed by people lightly
Because it is truly holy and powerful.

Chorus
They saw what they saw with their own eyes
And saw the strength and unity of the masses
And they firmly rejected being softened with words
They acted just the way they had always sworn they would.

Olenguruone masses saw with their own eyes,
Saw their cows and goats being penned away in kraals!
The children also witnessed Olenguruone being destroyed,
And all the wealth and hopes of the masses smashed.

They were herded into the colonial office
To have their fingerprints taken
They firmly refused to have their fingerprints taken
They were all detained in Yatta and in Nakuru
And all this because of their own own land.

Great were the cries among the Olenguruone children
Because of their suffering under torrential rains and horrible cold.
Children and mothers were crying together
Because their homes were burnt down.

Ngai saw the enemy destroy maize fields
He felt for the children suffering from hunger
And He blessed them with wild fruits and wild game
And He told them: 'Eat these to your fill.'

Schoolchildren were left alone in the yard
After their mothers and fathers were arrested
And taken to Yatta and Nakuru
And all because of their own own land.

Teacher Kaurugo was also arrested
But he firmly told the police:
'I will never leave the children orphaned
Meet me then at school
And they and I can go to jail together.'

Do not believe the enemy's deceptive words.
Never, never allow your fingerprints to be taken.
The justice of our cause and struggle
Is the covenant binding all African masses together.

When We Arrived at Olenguruone

When we came home to Olenguruone
We were tortured because of our land
We were told: 'Sign with your thumb-prints
So that you may have more land given to you.'
But they handed us court summons
So that we would leave them with our land.

Chorus
Say, say the trills and we go on trilling
As we the children of Mumbi are being evicted,
Thrown into lorries like logs,
Being tortured because of our land.

Our livestock and our food were auctioned
Great was the wailing, knowing as we did
That we had nothing to eat.
They destroyed maize plants in the fields
And they set fire to our houses.

We woke up early to unthatch the roofs and remove things
But if we were caught with the work unfinished
The houses would be burnt down.
We were packed into sheds like we were cattle
Then we would be removed from there
And be thrown into lorries.

And in the courtroom they would point guns at us
So that we would agree to sign away our lives
And if you refused to sign
You were given time in jail.

We were taken to Yatta Plains to die there
But Ngai said: 'No, I refuse to let it happen!'
We were given hardly any food
And were made to sweep and dig roads.

We were made to dig latrines naked
And if you refused to do so
You would have your rations cut!
They are making us suffer so because of our land
And to retard the liberation struggle of our country,
But we shall never give up our land and our freedom.

Yatta Detention Camp

There was great wailing in Olenguruone
Even as we collected together belongings
The enemy had scattered about.
The enemy was telling us:
Hurry up, quick!
Are you forgetting you are criminals?

Chorus
We will greatly rejoice
The day Kenyan people
Get back their land.

We left Olenguruone at four in the afternoon.
There were a lot of cattle at Cindarori
And many old men sorrowfully watched us
As we were being taken to detention.

We left Nakuru very early in the morning
And we arrived at Thika at noon.
For our breakfast they gave us
Three buckets of cold water.

The white settlers in Nairobi
Were rejoicing and laughing at us.
For they thought that
We were going to perish,
Never to return.

We met many people on the way to Yatta
Who told us: 'Go well, dear friends,'
In return we told them: 'Stay well, dear friends,
And know that we are going to the detention camp

In the land of "Mahiga Mairu" '[1]

We suffered a lot, oh, our people!
We were given *posho* full of worms.
We were brought to Yatta to perish
We were not brought here to live.

Gikuyu country has good arable land.
This land of Yatta is no good
It is full of black rocks and sand.

We were brought to Yatta to perish;
There is no rain, it is a desert.
We were brought here
Where there are no people
In order to destroy all hope in us.

We are being oppressed all over this land.
Even our homes have been destroyed
And our bodies have been exploited.
But do not be afraid
Because we are heading for a great victory.

The British came from Europe
In order to oppress our people
Since then they have continued oppressing us.
Ngai, when will they go back to Europe?

We shall continue to suffer for our freedom;
We shall continue struggling
For the return of our stolen land.
You British know that though you detain us
For demanding our land and freedom,
Kenya is ours for ever and ever.

Death of a Patriotic Woman

Women and children
Were singing praises to Kenyatta
While being taken to prison at Yatta

1. Black rocks.

Chorus
Pray truly, beseech him more
For Ngai is still the Ngai of old.

Three days and bitter tears
Dropped down our faces
After we saw the suffering of the children.
One woman died of a swollen stomach
After she had eaten the meat of a dead buffalo.

A white police officer came in the morning
Followed by his black lackeys carrying spades.
We saw them burying her like a beast,
But tears fell the moment
We saw with our own eyes
Her clothes being given to her sister.

A telephone call reached us from Githunguri
It was Jomo finding out
If we had arrived.
We told him of our great sorrow
Because of the death and burial of Josephine.

Great love I saw there among women and children:
If a bean fell to the ground,
They split it among themselves.
Bitter tears were shed by women and children
Because they were tormented
As they dug latrine pits.

The Cry of the Country

African people are now crying
Because they have been robbed of their land.
They now pause to ask:
'What is the people's future?'

Chorus
I ask: 'when will brave heroes be born?
To demand back our land without fear
Their hearts beating in unity!'

It is time you now looked with open eyes

And saw those who are supporting the British
Without remembering that
The property they once owned
Was taken from them without any reason!

Can't you think about the Olenguruone people,
How they were robbed of their wealth without reason
And their homes burnt down
And they were thrown out of their own land.

Oh, our people!
Have you so soon forgotten these things?
Is it because of selling your own souls
And our country to the foreign occupiers?
Can't you hear the cry of the country?

We know all the boundaries
Of all our land and country.
Do not allow yourselves to be deceived
By these imperialists from the race of the whites!

Better To Die Than To Sell Out The Country

Let us pray Mwene-nyaga
For the return of our land
Because it was taken from us
By the British colonialists.

Delamere swore and said that
He was all-powerful,
That he would remove Gikuyu
From the land they have occupied
To give room for the white settlers.

The white settlers told him:
'We will know you are all-powerful
When we see them
Moving out with their beehives and their children.'

Delamere brought a long train to Rongai
Which took many Gikuyu to Ndimu.
When we settled at Ndimu we were told
We could keep as many cattle on our small *shambas*.

After staying for three years on that land
We were told to reduce our livestock,
And our children were forced to work
On the settlers' estates.

Their work was to pick coffee-beans
Which were taken to Europe to enrich our oppressors.
A white man called 'Kihato' swore, saying that
He was power itself and he would take
The fingerprints of all the Agikuyu,
Then punish them.

He did not succeed because we resisted together
And we swore with all our might:
'It is better to die than to sell our country.'

We Shall Never Give Up

All our land, Kenyan people,
Was taken by foreigners,
And we and our children
Have persisted in crying.

Chorus
We shall never, never give up
Without land on which to grow food
And without our own true freedom
In our country of Kenya.

And that is why we were taken to detention
Because we were fighting for the future of our children
And we were taken to a desert place,
To this sandy wasteland.

And even if you keep silent or cry
We shall never stop making demands!
We shall be like our patriotic heroes,
Leaders of our nation.

Tears fell
The day we were taken to detention,
But Ngai gave us courage
Until we would be victorious!

There was great wailing among the children
Because of the pangs in their empty stomachs
For there was no milk to drink.

No, we shall never, never give up,
Without land on which to grow food
So that we provide for our children!

Women of Murang'a

We, the women of Murang'a were arrested
For refusing to have our goats and cattle poisoned.[2]
And because we rejected such colonial laws
We were thrown into prison cells
And our children were wailing
Because they had no milk to drink.

Chorus
We beseech you, our Ngai
Take us away from this slavery.

We were taken to Nairobi after being fingerprinted
And on the way they kept asking us:
'Do you belong to this conspiracy,
Fighting for Liberation?'
And our children continued wailing
Because they had no milk to drink.

The prison bosses came to the gate
To see these conspirators who are fighting for liberation.
And the children continued wailing
Because they had no milk to drink.

2. In early 1951 the British gave orders for Africans' cattle in Central Kenya to be inoculated against what they called 'rinderpest disease'. The result was that the cattle inoculated began dying en masse. In response, the peasants organized anti-inoculation demonstrations. Thousands of women from Murang'a stormed the inoculation centres – they burned down the cattle crushes and pens and chased away the inoculation operators. In retaliation, the forces of colonialism arrested more than 500 women and many others were hospitalized with serious injuries from police beatings. According to James Beauttah who was the KAU leader in Murang'a, the British were using the Africans' cattle as guinea-pigs to test their new vaccine. 'When we sent the vaccine secretly to London to be tested,' Beauttah explains, 'it was discovered that it was poisonous and could kill both cattle and people.'

Early in the morning
We saw porridge brought in a bucket,
There were no cups
So we drank out of pieces of broken pots.
And our children continued wailing
Because they had no milk to drink.

At eight in the morning
We saw many prison guards at the gate
Mercilessly they ordered us
To clean up the compound immediately.
And the children continued wailing
Because they had no milk to drink.

Detention of Dedan Mugo [3]

What do the Kenyan people think?
We did not sell our land,
The colonialists stole it from us.

I have been agitating
For the return of African land.
And I will never give up the struggle until victory.

Dedan Mugo, friend of the Africans,
Was detained by the colonialist enemy
For his commitment to the struggle
And his love for Kenya.

Dedan told the House of Mumbi:
'Never give up the struggle!
You must continue until my return.'

We did not invite you to Kenya,
You white oppressors.
Now you must go!
Leave Kenya — the black man's country!

3. The colonialists arrested Dedan Mugo wa Kimani in 1950 and sentenced him to
   five years in jail for being a member of the Mau Mau Movement. He was among the
   first Mau Mau casualties.

The 20th October 1952

It was late on the night of 20th October
When our national heroes were awakened
They were all arrested
And led to detention the same night
In the horror camps of the oppressors.

Chorus
There was much sorrow among those
Who were left behind:
Parents, children and friends were crying,
'Wuui, liya, Ngai help them
To come back to their homes safely.'

On the same night our leader was arrested
Surrounded by many police cars and weapons
He was told to carry only clothes in a suitcase.
He was not allowed to see his people
Or to say anything to them.

Each person had been arrested separately
With the police fully armed with weapons:
Rifles and pistols and clubs.
All the patriots were then assembled together that night.

When the patriots reached the detention camps
They were forced to sign thumb-prints on paper.
They were photographed, every patriot with a number.
The number had been made before the arrest.

A Letter from Prison

When I was at home I had many friends,
But when I went to prison they all abandoned me.
That is why those who are not committed to the cause
Cannot be trusted at all.

We agreed that I would find them waiting for me,
What happened to make them deceive me?
They will realize that jail is not death
And I will surely return home.

My prison term will be over, dear mother,
I implore Ngai to return me home safely,
To see each other with our own eyes
So you can truly believe that I'm still alive,
And I shall die when Ngai wills!

When I am led to the quarry by the warders
Pick-axe on the shoulder,
Karai[4] on the head
The warders often pray that their jobs
Last for many more years to come,
But me, I pray: 'Return me home soon!'

The half-cooked *posho* we eat, dear mother,
Is wrapped in a dirty rag like a dead body,
But we dared not refuse it,
Ngai is great,
We will surely return home.

If you glanced inside
Through the prison gates, dear mother,
You cannot find a European or an Asian —
Only us the children of the soil being tortured.

The Song of Prison

Comrades, let us sing this song of sorrow
Which we used to sing
When we were in prison.

Chorus
We used to leave the prison gate in twos!
We had to raise high our clothes for search
On our way to labour.

The food we ate was wrapped
In a dirty piece of cloth
And was carried in a coffin
Like a dead body.

4. A metal basin used by prisoners to carry concrete.

Some of my friends deserted me
When I was jailed.
When one is jailed for good deeds
He is detested by some.

Very early in the morning before daybreak
The trumpet was blown for us to wake up
And wrap up our beddings.

There was much suffering inside the jail.
The stinking buckets used for latrines
Were at the foot of our beds.

The type of work we did
During our imprisonment
Was to carry heavy stone building blocks.

There was much suffering because
If one did not fulfil his quota,
Whether sick or dying,
He was not allowed to eat for that day.

Let us all embrace and shake hands
Because Ngai has helped us
And we have come back to our homes.

Prisons Are Terrible Places

Prisons are terrible places
They have swallowed all our sons.
But parents, rejoice now,
For Ngai is great,
Those who survived the prisons have returned.

The traitors of the land are worthless animals:
They betrayed us
They had us arrested
They had us put into prison;
But Ngai is great, we shall come back.

All African people in this country
Should resist without ceasing
Until our patriots win the struggle;

When they win we will regain our freedom.

When our patriotic forces win the struggle
Where will you traitors,
The barren of the land, run to?
For you have betrayed us
And caused us to suffer terribly;
Ngai is with us, we shall be free.

Story of Kamiti Prison

In Kamiti there was a traitorous wardress
Whose name was Waithira.
She forced our children to remain behind
So that she could have them poisoned.

When we left for work
Our children were taken to Cecelia[5]
Who administered the poison
In medicines and injections.

Traitor Waithira was always happy
To see so many of our children dying.
She usually woke up very early
To count the number of the dead.

Oh, our people!
We lost many children at Kamiti
Especially during the month of July.
Mostly it was boys who died.

Traitor Waithira are you aware that
It is the children of the Mau Mau patriots
Who you are murdering by giving them poison?
You will pay with your life.

5. A Briton in charge of the prison clinic.

We Oppose Foreign Domination

A lot of discussion and happiness
Ended with my detention.
I shall remember all this after my release.
Wuui, take me home to Gikuyuland,
A beautiful and fertile land,
Belonging to my forefathers.

Our eyes are full of tears,
Our hearts are heavy,
Wuui, take me back home,
A beautiful and fertile land,
Belonging to Mumbi.

Our old defence walls are collapsing,
Though we have put up a hard fight.
You must now fully prepare yourselves.
This is a continuous war.

You traitors to our cause,
You are the real problem.
Why can't you be guided
By hearts' devotion to our noble cause?

When your hero arrived from India,[6]
You were all summoned to Githunguri
For a grand celebration.

At a meeting in Nakuru, Koinange declared:
'We will never accept to be ruled by foreigners,
Better for us all to die.'

After the meeting the cowards
Tried to join the people,
They were laughed at by the children
And were even hated by their colonial masters.

6. Refers to James Beauttah who, in 1947, went to India to attend the All-Asian Conference.

The Story of the Struggle in Kisii

Nine thousand and ninety-nine of us
Were summoned to Kisii town
When we arrived there
We found a large group of people.

The enemies of the Gikuyu said:
'Any person who calls himself a Gikuyu
Should be eliminated so that he will never claim
That he is the owner of the country.'

After they had finished talking,
There then came a white mercenary
Followed by Blacklegs
Who surrounded the children of Mumbi.

After that those who sided
With the British came forward
And loudly announced that
They didn't want to die for an independence which,
They were sure, would never come.
And the enemies clapped for them.

After they had clapped they then led us
To the torture chambers
Where they had dug a deep trench with spikes.
And they would throw us there to be spiked.

Ngai, the all-powerful, helped us.
We were not injured by the spikes
Only three persons were spiked
And their wounds were deep and serious.

Those who denounced us
Went back to our homes afterwards
To maltreat our women and children
And to loot all the property
We had left behind.

Only one question that each should ask of himself:
What is the benefit of giving away the children,
For their bodies to be meals for lions?

The Wind and the Sun

In the fabled argument between the wind and the sun
Each claims to be the most powerful.
Even after sun defeated wind,
They continued struggling to this day.

Chorus
When I cross the cold river
Looking to the East
I will be happy with all my heart
And I'll keep on praising the leader.

The fight between Kisii Home Guards and Gikuyu
Started at Kisii town.
Because of being deceived by our enemies,
They told us to leave.

And you our elders remain patient
And return your children to the East.
A hungry person does not choose his food
He can even eat an antelope
Though it is very tough.

Children of other nationalities
Remain in peace.
Now we are returning to the East
Where Ngai gave land to Gikuyu and Mumbi
For them to live there for ever and ever.

The Sufferings of Kenyan Patriots

Whose child is this
Lying by the fireside crying?

Chorus
If I am called by Kimathi
I will go
He is our leader
He is our liberator
Let us embrace him.

Who is this being tortured

And yet remains a great patriot?

And who is this weeping
Because whites are being driven out of Kenya?

At Embakasi in broad daylight!
Who is being tortured?

Who is this you are torturing?
He is the leader of the Black people.

And won't he be a great hero?
He who defeats British colonialism?

Who are the foreigners,
Who exploit this country?

And you who now sell us to foreigners,
Where will you go when the whites are driven out?

Home Guards Will Pay for their Treachery

On January 7th we were surrounded at Bahati
By the forces of colonialism.

Chorus
We shall never be silent
Until we get enough land to cultivate
And Freedom in this our Country of Kenya.

Home Guards, the traitors, were the first to come
And close the gates.
Then the British mercenary troops entered
While the police surrounded the location.

We were ordered out of our houses
And told to pack up our belongings
As we were to be detained.

We packed our things
And then they took us to an open field
Where many Gikuyu and other nationalities
Were selected for detention.

69

Some of those chosen were taken to Manyani,
Others to Mackinnon Road,
Where they met untold suffering.

You traitors!
You only care for your stomachs
You are the enemies of our people
You shall pay for your treachery with your life
When we seize our freedom.

Embakasi Detention Camp

We were taken to Langata Detention camp
On the 22nd day of April,
Where we joined others
Who were arrested before us.

As we passed through the gate
A British Police Officer enquired
Whether we were members of the Movement
That was fighting for Independence.

Speaking with heroism and confidence
We firmly answered:
'Yes, we are!
And we will fight to the end.'

We stayed in Langata for three days
On the fourth day we were lined up at the gate
Where we found traitor Wanjau
And his clique of Gakonias[7] awaiting us.
He ordered that we be physically searched.
With our faces covered they put us into lorries
Which took us to Embakasi Camp.

On our arrival at Embakasi
Traitor Wanjau gave orders that we be beaten.
After the savage beatings
Each of us was supplied
With yellow pants and black shirts.

7. See Appendix.

On the back of the shirts
Was written in capital letters:
HARDCORE MAU MAU.

After a fortnight's stay
Nine of our comrades
Were taken to the torture chamber
Where they were mercilessly tortured,
But none of them agreed to surrender.
They firmly told their sadistic torturers:
'We would rather die than give up our country!'

Three days later
Nine more of our comrades
Were dragged into the torture room.
Except Kamau who broke down and surrendered
The rest of the comrades
Stood firmly by their convictions.

On the evening of the tenth day of May
After our daily chores
We were summoned before the colonialist
In charge of the camp.
With him there were three traitors including Kamau
Who identified the leaders of our group.

After our leaders were taken away
The sadistic colonialist gave us a long lecture,
Threatening us that if we don't surrender
And denounce the Movement
He would make us suffer.

Collectively, but firmly, we told him:
'We shall never surrender
And we are ready to die for our country!'
As a result he gave orders
That we be locked in
Without food or water for three days.
In agreement the traitors clapped.

Mackinnon Road Detention Camp

We left Murang'a at six in the morning.
There were children and women
Who sorrowfully watched us
As we were taken to detention.

We arrived at Thika about eight.
For our breakfast they gave us
Three buckets of cold porridge;
We refused to drink it.

In order to force us to drink it,
Traitor 'Speaker'[8] gave orders
That we be beaten:
Many of us were seriously injured,
Two of our comrades died.

On our arrival at Langata Detention Camp
We were ordered to take off our clothes.
Then traitor 'Speaker' gave orders
That we be beaten again.
Oh, our people, we suffered a great deal.

While we were still naked
They rushed us to compound Number 21
Leaving our belongings behind.
They were brought to us two hours later.

When we reached the compound
We were told to squat in lines
Each containing eight people,
And to place our hands on the top of our heads.

We were ordered to sing loud;
'Mau Mau Mbaya'.[9]
When we firmly refused to do so,
In spite of the blows from their clubs,
They ordered us to lie on our stomachs naked
In the mud
As they continued beating us.

8. This traitor baptized himself as 'Speaker'.
9. Broken Swahili meaning, 'Mau Mau is bad.'

The following day early in the morning
We were ordered to line up
In the front of five Gakonias
Who identified and pronounced
Some of us Hardcore Mau Mau.

After three days in Langata
We were lined up at our compound gate.
They loaded us into the lorries
Which took us to the Railway Station.
We were on our way to Mackinnon Road.

On the fourth day of September 1954
We arrived at Mackinnon Road Detention Camp.
They took us to a place near the kitchens
Where we were to be searched.
We were ordered to remove all our clothes:
They took all our belongings
And we were allowed to remain
With only one set of clothes.

The next morning the traitors were brought in
To identify the real Mau Mau Hardcores among us.
We were all classified as Hardcores
And sent to compound Number 9
Where we had to endure
Many brutal tortures for five years.

Our compatriots,
The struggle will be long
And fraught with suffering and death.
But whatever sacrifices we have to make
And however long the struggle will last
Our determination is to fight to the end
Until we get back our land and African freedom.

Our Journey to Lamu Detention Camp

We endured untold suffering
On the journey to Lamu detention camp.
It took us three days to reach there.

Chorus
Whether we are tortured
Or deported to remote islands
We shall never cease to agitate
For the return of our land
And freedom for our country.

Carrying our belongings on our shoulders
We were put on a train at Maboko around eight at night,
But none of us showed any fear.

We met many Kenyans at Mariakani
Who were brought there by the colonialists
To see us, 'the evil Mau Mau gangsters'.
We were forced out of the train and paraded
So that they could see and mock us.

Secretly, but firmly, we told these Kenyans
That they should not accept colonial propaganda,[10]
And that we were patriots fighting
For Kenya's independence.
Then we were loaded on lorries
And taken on to Malindi.

In Malindi we suffered terribly
We were packed into small box-cells
Where we could hardly breathe.
Some died from suffocation.

At Rangola Simba Forest we met our comrades
Who were detained there,
We embraced each other with joy.
They gave us food and a place to sleep.

On our way to Lamu
We experienced all kinds of sufferings:
Daily hunger and severe beatings,

10. As the Movement began to spread among other nationalities, the colonialists started
a propaganda programme amongst the non-Gikuyu, Embu and Meru nationalities.
Their aims were twofold: to recruit them into their terrorist army and to divide the
Kenyan masses by propagating tribalism, by claiming mainly that Mau Mau was not
a national movement. One notorious part of this fascist programme was to make a
public parade of some hungry, tortured and chained prisoners of war. The spectators
were told that Mau Mau guerrillas ate people and that they lived in forests like wild
animals. In such parades there were some Kenyan traitors who jeered and mocked
at the patriots.

Heavy rains and disease.

We were taken to Lamu by boat.
On our arrival we were locked up
In those old dungeons Arabs used
To keep our people during the slave trade.

After a few days hundreds more of our people
Were brought to the island
Where we had to endure
All kinds of tortures for seven years.

The traitors who opposed our liberation struggle
Were brought to the island to torture us.
They mocked us saying:
'Look at these fools
Who will be struggling till eternity.'

Our Struggle in Tanganyika

We were very happy
When we arrived in Tanganyika
Because we met our compatriots
Who lived there.

We suffered a great deal during our stay there
From British oppression
And some of us were deported to Kenya.[11]

In order to get our means of life
We were kept as squatters.
The working conditions were extremely oppressive;
Some of us died.

After staying on the plantation for two years,
We received orders:

11. In order to combat the spread of Mau Mau in Tanganyika, the colonial regime
declared a state of emergency in the Northern region (Kilimanjaro and Meru areas)
in 1953, All Kenyan nationals in the country, particularly the Gikuyu, Embu, Meru
and Kamba nationalities, were arrested and deported back to Kenya. Those who
were identified as members of the Movement were tortured and then jailed; some
were murdered outright.

Once our crops had germinated and started to grow
We must all have our fingerprints taken.

On November the 4th 1951,
They told us to get fingerprinted
Or else they would deport us back to Kenya.

When these cruel orders were read to us
Our first reaction was to ask guidance from Ngai
And he showed us the path of resistance,
We decided to go on strike!

The Labour Officer to whom we took our complaints
Was in league with our colonial enemy;
Instead of helping us he only added
To our suffering and bitterness.

On the 9th in a detention camp in the town,
We were very sad because our attempt
To sell our grain before leaving
The plantation was frustrated.
Our grain was thrown out in the streets.

On December the 5th 1951, some among us
Who were politically weak, broke down
And surrendered to the enemy.
They agreed to be fingerprinted.

But, we, the majority refused to be fingerprinted
We persisted with the resistance
And they deported us back to Kenya.

Song of Africa [12]

Ngai gave to Black people
This land of Africa
Which abounds in fertile soil and good streams.
Praise the Ngai who dwells in High Places

12. This patriotic song was composed by our people in the detention camp to commemorate the Independence of Ghana. It is clear from the song that our people saw the liberation struggle in our country as an integral part of the liberation struggle of the whole continent of Africa.

Because of His love for us.

Chorus
We will ever continue to praise
The land of Africa
From East to West
From North to South.

After much suffering
Egypt freed herself from slavery
And she got back her freedom.

And when Ethiopia saw light
Shining down from the East
She struggled very hard
And she freed herself
From the mud of slavery.

We were very happy
When we heard that Ghana was free
That she had hauled down the British flag.

If you look around the whole of Kenya
You will see one river of blood
Because the general aim is one:
To get back our freedom.

Listen to the general cry
Of our brothers in South Africa
Where they continue to be oppressed
By the racist Boers.

We shall be very very happy
When all the Black people come together
So that we forge in unity
One Pan-African state.

PART 3
Guerrilla Songs

Let us make this very clear: If one of the KAU leaders or
anybody else gets in our way, we will cut him down just the
same we have done to those who stood in our way.

Kimathi's Papers

When we say *Comrades* we are using a word bathed in
blood and sacrifices. Comrades are those who have fought
in clandestinity, those who suffered torture and death in
the prisons, those who gave of their bodies and intellect
on the battlefield, those who built freedom, those who
made us what we are, those capable of translating their
aspirations into action, who have devoted their lives to the
service of our people.

Samora Machel
The Tasks Ahead

I did not know how to bear it, and for days and weeks I
hobbled about with the same song in my head: So they had
killed my family and I alone was left . . . Then I recalled
that Kimathi had lost his brothers and that his mother had
gone crazy and that he himself was later killed and all this
for the sake of our struggle.

Ngugi wa Thiong'o
Petals of Blood

And nothing is more in accordance with human dignity
than to die fighting for the liberation of one's country from
foreign domination.

Viet Nam Courier

Our Leader, Dedan Kimathi

When our Kimathi ascended
Into the mountains alone
He asked for strength and courage
To decisively defeat the colonialists.

He said that we should tread
The paths that he had trodden,
That we should follow his revolutionary footsteps
And drink from his cup.

If you drink from the cup of courage,
That cup I have drunk from myself,
It is a cup of pain and of suffering,
A cup of tears and of death.

We are tortured because we are Black;
We are not white people
And we are not of their kind.
But with Ngai in us
We shall defeat the colonialists.

Do not be afraid of imprisonment
Nor should you lose heart for being detained.
Even when they confiscate our property
And kill us
Do not ever despair:
Because of our faith and commitment
We shall defeat the enemy.

You must take his courage and endurance
To courageously face tribulations or death,
Knowing that you will belong
To the Black people's state of Kenya.

Declaration of War in Kenya

When the war was declared in 1952
Our country was turned into a huge prison.
Innocent people, men, women and children,
Were herded into concentration camps,
Under all kinds of harsh repression.

Kenyan patriots were arrested and killed,
Thousands of others were subjected
To slow death in Manyani
And Mackinnon Road concentration camps.

KAU leaders were arrested
And taken to Kapenguria
Where they faced a Kangaroo court.

Large-scale massacres of our people
Were committed across the country.
Meanwhile Kimathi in Nyandarwa called for total mobilization,
He told the people to unite and fight
These foreign murderers with heroism
And drive them out of the country.

Our Independent Schools, the people's schools,
Were turned into gallows
Where many of our compatriots
Experienced untold suffering and death.

Our livestock were confiscated
And our crops in the fields were destroyed.
All public markets were closed down
And all people's newspapers were banned.

Thousands of patriotic women
Were locked in prisons.
Many of them, with their children,
Were put into concentration camps
Where they suffered all kinds of brutal tortures.

Later the colonialists employed
Vast numbers of Kenyans who took up rifles
To fight as mercenaries in opposition to the Motherland,
To kill and torture their own compatriots
Leaving behind countless widows and orphans.

In spite of harsh enemy repression,
The revolutionary flame was maintained and developed.
And people's hatred toward the British oppressors
Grew from day by day,
And proudly they declared:
'It would be better to die on our feet
Than to live on our knees.'

They Were Sitting In Nyandarwa

They were sitting in Nyandarwa
The shepherds of the masses
Preparing the strategy
How to fight the colonialists.

When Kimathi finished talking
Mbaria stood up and said:
'We shall fight until victory!'

General Kariba
Together with General Tanganyika
Have been sent to Mount Kenya
To lead our guerrilla army there.

He has been born today,
The Commander-in-Chief of our army.
He has been born in Nyandarwa
The cultivator of Justice.

When Gitau was captured
He never panicked,
He said that he was very happy
So that the prophesy can be fulfilled.

Even if you detained all of us
You will never win
Since we have a great hero
And he lives in Nyandarwa.

Though you banned both KCA and KAU
You did not succeed
Since we have already formed another one
And it is called Mau Mau.

Unity and cooperation are demanded from you,
You the Mau Mau members,
So that we can fight for our land together.

The Decisive Moment in Our Struggle

Many people will weep with joy
When Kimathi comes
With Kenya's Independence.

Chorus
Those who have faith in the struggle
Will rejoice when Kimathi comes
Bringing Kenya's Independence.

He will not come as powerless as before,
He will come with power,
And with great faith in the masses
He will make his political base at Kianyandarwa.
And the House of Mumbi and all Kenya's nationalities
Will be freed from slavery forever.

We will rejoice together
When we get our freedom
Which has caused so many of us
To be detained and others to be imprisoned.
Those who betrayed us,
Where will they run to?

He asks the young men and women:
Who are the stronger,
You or the elders?
Our land was taken from them
Without much resistance,
And if you don't fight for it now
Whom will you blame?

This is the decisive moment
For the Kenyan masses
We must fight hard to get our land back
Because if we delay there will be others
Who will come pretending to be our friends
But they will be our great enemies.
They too will take our land
And we shall have a difficult time getting it back.

Rise Up, You Youth

Rise up, you youth.
The masses are calling you.
Arm yourselves with spears and shields
Do not delay, come quickly,
Come help the masses.
The enemy is British colonialism
And it is very vicious.

Rise up, you youth.
It is time for war.
Forget your drinking
Take up arms.
Those who are armed
And committed to the cause
Can never be defeated.

Rise up, you youth.
The war is on.
You will win because Ngai is in us.
Rise up! Don't be afraid.
Armed with discipline,
Armed with faith and commitment
You will definitely win.

We are fighting for our land.
Yet some of our people
Don't seem to understand
The root causes of our struggle.
Can't they see that we are oppressed
Because of agitating for our Independence
And full rights to our land?

Those who haven't joined the people's Movement
Should be informed about it,
And that we are waiting for them to join.
Come immediately to fight for our land
Which was taken by the colonialists by force
Reducing us to beggars in our own country.

The People's Soldiers

The soldiers of our nation
Are all the African people of Kenya.

Beautiful, beautiful people in unity!
To defend what we inherited from our ancestors,
Ngai in us,
We will triumph.

The railway line has reached to the Great Lake
As foreseen by the old prophets.
Now you whites must realize
We shall drive you into the sea.

Kenyan people, take up the leadership!
Wake up all those who are now asleep.
We must be at one with our fighters
For they will surely bring our liberation.

We Will Smash Their Political Power

Now the enemy does not sleep
For thinking how he can destroy
Our national liberation movement.

Wake up the youth!
Seize the leadership from the elders,
Because if you hesitate, the foreign enemy
Will seize more of our land and wealth.

In the fifty-two years of colonialism
All of us can see how terribly we have suffered,
And how some of our people have collaborated
With the colonialists to oppress us.

Why betray our country for money?
Is a thousand shillings equal to our country?
What will you do when it is finished?
The colonialists will abandon you,
Where then will you run to?

We cannot allow these foreigners to remain here

While they continue to suck our blood.
We will smash their political power
And throw them out of the country.
This is our country
We have the right to rule ourselves.

Seize the Time

Our people, we are in great danger!
And we are in for a lot of trouble,
But understand that it is only through struggle
Through our own strength and courage
That we can overcome all this
And seize our national freedom.

And you who are sleeping
Wake up now!
Follow the revolutionary path of the people
Remember that only through unity in struggle
Shall we be able to liberate our land.

Seize the time!
Make haste how!
Join the struggle for land
And never betray the African people.

Don't think you are a patriot
When you join the enemy forces.
Remember that to betray your people
Is an act of treason.

I Am Not Afraid, I Must Go

I am not afraid, I must go
I must go and fight for our country.

Chorus
I will fight the enemy!
I will fight the enemy!
I will tell him:

'Go your way, leave our land!'

White enemies will come
And I will not be afraid.
Holding the shield of justice and truth,
I will wipe them out.

This land has been ours
Since time immemorial
And all its riches belong to us.

You traitors of the land
You should realize that this country
Belongs to Black people
And it will be ours forever.

When you sing this song
Try to understand how serious it is,
It is a song of sorrow and suffering.

Rise and Take Up Arms

Waiyaki died a long time ago,
And even then
He was struggling so that our country
May not be taken by the foreign invaders.

Waiyaki was tortured
That time, a long time back,
Struggling for our country
So that we could find some shelter.

After Waiyaki was arrested
He prayed to Ngai
That other fighters would rise
Who would continue the struggle for the land.

Masses all over the country,
Now listen:
The hero who has been sent by Ngai
Is Dedan Kimathi.

Oh, our people,

For what did you send Kimathi to the forest?
What was he to get from out there?
It was so that he would liberate us
From white colonialists.

The masses of this land
Listen to and follow Kimathi
Because he would like us to unite
And fight for the land to be returned.

If you fail to get his message
You will be corrupted by the whites
And you will start whispering
Treacherous words by night
Thus selling your people to the whites.

Don't listen to the whites
Because they will surely return to their homes.
Those who have accepted fingerprinting
Are their true slaves.

Those who fawn
On these British oppressors,
They should remember
They will one day go away.
Where will traitors then run to?

Victoriously we shall all gather together
We the Kenyan people
To celebrate our birthright in dance and song.

The Fountain of Independence

The fountain of our Independence
Sprang from Kimathi
And he said it would be guarded by the Mau Mau army
And it would be protected with stones erected around it.
We shall destroy you, the whites,
Because you only know robbery and violence.

All the whites who are here
Are now in great danger:
The Mau Mau forces will destroy you.

The Kenyan masses will sit in judgement over you
And they will order you to go back to your country.
We shall destroy you, the whites,
Because you only know robbery and violence.

You whites must know that you will leave this country
Because this is not your country.
You came here to rob and oppress us
It is time you went back to Europe.
Then only Black people will be left here
To enjoy the fruits of their toil
And rights to their land.

Those with hearts of steel were made so by Kimathi
He recruited Kago and then sent him to Nyandarwa
To fight for our liberation.
We shall destroy you, the whites,
Because you only know robbery and violence.

Kimathi, Save Us from Slavery

Good Ngai who supports our national army,
Who kindly receives African people's sacrifices,
As long as you are our guide
The enemy cannot defeat us.

We pray to you with love and respect
And with patriotic feelings,
And with unity in our struggle.
With you in us we shall drive the foreigners out.

Go quickly Kimathi
And save us from this slavery.
Kenya is filled with bitter tears
Struggling for liberation.

Remember that the white colonialists hate us.
They hunt us day and night
Their aim is to exterminate us all.

Mau Mau is preaching love and unity in struggle.
If you want to share patriotic love
Join Mau Mau without delay.

Go now Kimathi!
Bring us Independence
Kenya is filled with bitter tears
Struggling for our liberation.

Kimathi Will Bring Our National Anthem

Kimathi will bring our national anthem
Along with a flag of liberation from Nyandarwa
When we seize back our freedom.

Because we are true members of the Movement
We will arm ourselves
And firmly tell the British oppressors to leave.

You shall see our people
Who have so long been oppressed
Seizing independence under Kimathi.

Kimathi will identify
Those who have been oppressing us
And the British will be driven out,
Together with their African puppets.

Those of our people
Who have been oppressing us
Will be thrown into the bonfire
Because they collaborated with the British
And helped them steal our land.

They will be asked by our people:
'Because you were deceived by the British
And sold our land,
Why don't you follow them now?'

We, the African people of Kenya,
Will all rejoice when our land
Which was sold
By those who wanted to be chiefs
Is returned to us.

You White People Are Foreigners in Our Country

You white people,
You are foreigners in our country.
You brought slavery and exploitation to our country.
Now leave our country!
You are foreigners.

Chorus
I will fight our enemy
I will fight our enemy
Until our country is free.

Ngai gave us this land
And he gave you yours in Britain,
Why then did you come to our country
To steal our land?
You are foreigners in this country.

And you traitors
Who sell us to the white oppressors
You must realize that
We will expel the white oppressors
From this our land.
Then you will pay
For your treacherous acts with your lives.

You who sell us are our great enemies!
Look around you and look at the whites
And also look at yourselves.
The whites are foreigners,
And they will surely go back to their country,
Where will you, traitors to your country, run to?

Kenya Is Our Inheritance

We salute all of you parents
With happiness and great joy,
Because Ngai has made possible for us
To meet again in happiness.

Chorus
Agitate! Agitate! Agitate!

For the return of our land.

The heroes of our Army,
Kimathi and Mathenge, fight hard
To rid Kenya of white racists
And free our parents from sorrow.

This country of ours,
Rich with fertile soil,
Belongs to the Kenyan people,
It is their birthright.

The elders of Mwangi and Irungu generations
May Ngai enable them
To remain united and loving
'Ta gikwa na mukungugu.'[1]

Remember the old proverb, which says:
'He who works hard never goes unhelped.'
'The child of a good home does not eat rubbish.'
May the beloved patriot beget those who will listen.

Kenya is our land by inheritance
It is our natural right
Where we graze goats and cattle,
But the foreigners
Have taken all of our land
Now we have no place to graze.

In the Garden Were Many Fruits

In the garden were many fruits!
With my love, Josephine Njeri,
Drinking and eating together,
I never thought we would part.

I asked for a hundred shillings
From my father for solving my marriage problems,
My father refused all that!
And all that is my own heart's pain.

1. A Gikuyu metaphor meaning literally 'as a yam vine is to the tree that props it up'.

One's own mother is the only one
Who feels with one:
If the woman who had given birth to me was alive
I would not have gone to sleep without that money
To solve my marriage problems.

On the 8th of September
I wept my eyes dry
Because of my love,
Her name was Njeri.

I am sad because Njeri is pregnant
And I don't know what the elders will say
Look after all that, my Ngai
Because I am an orphan.

Now stay in peace my love
I am going deep into the forest
To fight for the land and freedom of the Kenyans.

The House of Mumbi has no enmity with anybody
And it never thinks of creating enmity with anybody.
He who hates it, may he be cursed by Ngai
He who loves it, may he be kept well by Ngai.

When I Married Njoki

When I married Njoki I did not think
She was a good woman, better than Nyambura.
On returning home from work
I would always find my food on the table,
My clothes washed,
I was always filled with happiness.

But Nyambura loved me and I too loved her.
There is no doubt or obstacle
Nyambura, we shall surely marry.

After we were seven months in the forest
Nyambura told me: 'I now must go to see my mother,
I will return to your home
When you leave the forest.'

When I heard that,
I started on my feet toward her parents' home
So I would get back my bridewealth to marry another;
I don't want Nyambura anymore!

When Nyambura heard that she started weeping.
I told her: 'Nyambura, stop weeping!
I am not to blame, you are to blame,
So wipe off your tears.'

Nyambura, goodbye,
I am going back to the forest
I'll only come back here after Uhuru is achieved
And when we get back our land.

Will You Persevere Through Death?

The children of Gikuyu live in the forest
Soaking wet in the pouring rains
Hungry and cold and suffering
For the love of their soil.

Chorus
Uui, Uui, Uui, iiyai!
Will you persevere through death, jail
And continuous sufferings and misery?

Who are those singing aloud
Across the other side of the river,
Praising Kago and Mbaria, our Generals,
Seekers of freedom and justice?

Some amongst us have betrayed us
To the British oppressors.
They sold us out for money
Because they thought we would never win
But we have won.

Police Harrassment

In Nairobi I am harrassed by the occupying forces
And if I return to the countryside
I am a Mau Mau 'gangster'.

Chorus
What shall I do?
What shall I do?
To be free from this slavery?

I'll pay any price
For the light of liberation,
And when it comes
I will live in dignity.

We must struggle together as one people.
Let us all unite
And become like the foundation stone.

You traitors selling our people
For personal power,
Remember that Kenyan people forever condemn you!

The composer of this song
Is a Mau Mau cadre.
He suffered greatly in detention camps.

The Home Guards Destroyed Our Homes

I left home,
Promising my parents and friends that
I was going to the forest
To fight for the land
And freedom for African people.

Chorus
Follow the young man
And remember
This soil is ours.

The hero you see
With a gap between the teeth

Is called Ndungu wa Gaceru.
He shoots down enemy's warplanes
When they come to harass *itungati*[2] in Nyandarwa.

Manyeki Wang'ombe,
The hero of Murang'a,
Gave his own life
For the liberation of this country.

When I went home from the forest
I found my parents sleeping in the rain.
Weeping they said: 'Oh, our dear son,
The home guards burned our houses.'

Mother, whether you cry or not,
I will only come back
When we get our land back and African freedom.

We Will Finally Triumph

As we part with each other, comrades,
Remember that it is only our bodies that part.
Our spirits, our hearts, go together.

Chorus
If you are asked
Whether you are an African
Firmly lift your two hands high
And assert categorically
You are an African!

When we part, comrades,
And go to our homes
Each with greetings and love to the parents
And to brothers and sisters.

When I get home
I will dress in ancestral skin robes
Wash my face and smear myself with oil,
There will be love and rejoicing all over Gikuyuland.

2. See Appendix.

Once again we call all young men
To serve the masses with dedication
For, despite the persecutions,
We will finally triumph.

The call also goes to the women
To unite with their men
To defeat the cunning colonialists,
They and their offspring.

Our Journey to Nyandarwa

Marira turned to, and demanded of, Commander Chotara:
'Why did you order us to remain in Nairobi
Knowing very well that
Our comrades have left for Nyandarwa?'

And Commander Chotara replied:
'Pack all your things now
Because tomorrow we will travel to Nyandarwa.'

The guerrillas were happy
They packed up their things quickly,
Happily saying: 'We now go
To fight for our people's freedom.'

And you, our dear parents, do not fear:
It is known a baby can die soon after birth
And its parents will endure the pain,
Knowing the cause of the death.

When we reached Kandara
We spotted the enemy forces.
General Kago declared:
'We shall engage them in battle
No Iregi warrior was ever afraid of death.'

When we reached Nyandarwa Headquarters
Kimathi was very happy to see us,
He said: 'You have arrived in triumph,
Brave patriots of the land.'

June the 5th we left Mbaria's unit

Heading for Tuthu to see our guerrilla comrades
And when we arrived at Mathioya River
We found many difficulties:
Rain, cold, mud
And hunger throughout the night.

In the forest we lived through more difficulties:
Death, heavy rains and many days of hunger;
Snow and frost had become our food.
But despite these difficulties
We will definitely triumph.

Follow Behind the Youth

When I returned to Gikuyuland I was shocked
My parents were now homeless and miserable
They said tearfully: 'Oh, son
Our homes were burned down.'

Chorus
Follow behind the youth
And remember
This country is forever ours!

Goodbye and peace be with you,
Dear parents and friends,
I am going back to Nyandarwa
To fight for freedom.
I am committed to the liberation of Kenyan people,
Praise be to Mwene-Nyaga.

When I returned to the forest
I found the comrades safe and well.
As comrades-in-arms we embraced one another with joy.
We are committed to the liberation of Kenyan people.
Praise be to Mwene-Nyaga.

We Are Born Here

When we arrived in Location 10[3]
The peasants gave us food
And slaughtered a ram,
For rations on our mission.

Chorus
We were happy as we went
We were happy as we returned
Because our mission was a victory both ways.

When we arrived at Rwathia Githioro
The enemy forces surrounded us,
General Ihuura commanded boldly:
'Put your guns in position
And be ready to fight.'

Ihuura, you are a great patriot.
Get rid of the white man
So that we have peace in the country.

When we arrived at Gaicanjiru
We were welcomed by our Akamba contacts
They cautioned us not to sleep there
Because the area was occupied by the home guards.

Gitau replied boldly:
'We are going to sleep here,
This is where we were born!'

The Song of Gitau Matenjagwo

Gitau Matenjagwo,
The sole one I know from Muthithi to Kariara.
That is him you see in the picture, a patriot
Busy serving his people.

The braves we sent to the Ndakaini battle
Were Kimathi and Mbaria,

3. Refers to Weithaga Location in Murang'a District.

They fought so courageously
And with such great dedication
That all the guerrillas
Were filled with joy.

The one lying down in the picture
Is Kago wa Mboko
He shoots down the enemy warplanes
That harass and bomb Murang'a.

Gitau told Wamwere, the betrayer:
'Wamwere don't betray me,
Wamwere don't betray me,
If you are a true son of the land.'

Wamwere replied:
'Come get him!
He is here!
He tells me not to betray him
So that our homes can be burnt.'

Just before his death
Gitau Matenjagwo put a handful of soil
In his mouth
And with his clenched fist held skyward,
He said: 'I am dying as an African hero.'

Kiiru the Killer

Continue sleeping.
When Kiiru[4] comes
I will wake you up.

Continue sleeping.
If he comes
I will let you know.

I will sleep no more.

---

4. Henry Kiiru was a colonial chief in Kiru Location, Murang'a, during the Mau Mau war of national liberation. Before he was eliminated, he had killed more than a hundred people. His death was celebrated in the whole district by our people.

Otherwise he will find me sleeping
When he comes.

A special order came from Nyandarwa
That Kiiru must be eliminated.

You home guard traitors should all be dead
And get lost forever.
Why do you continue killing us
When we are fighting for our land
And freedom for all of us?

Throughout this region
I only know Kago wa Mboko
The Commander of the Mau Mau forces in Murang'a.

Youth of Nairobi

Youth of the town,
You are very happy for making love
While the guerrillas are in the forest.

We saw the home guards running at us
With their shot-guns ready,
But we were not afraid
Because we were the heroes of the people.

You *'taitai'* should know that
You sold us out for money
While Kimathi is in the forest
Fighting for our land and freedom.

As the country's heroes
We have won the war
And you traitors who sold us for money,
What will become of you?

Kimathi's letter came from Nyandarwa.
He was concerned with our revolutionary work in Nairobi
And our failures to wipe out Henderson's *'taitai'* force.

In our reply we expressed our concern
Because many of our comrades

Had been detained during Operation Anvil[5]
While others were being tortured at Embakasi.[6]

Youth of Nairobi fight with courage
We will get our freedom
And our land will be returned.

Kimathi's Wife Was the Secretary

One of our women contacts brought a message:
'Enemy forces are coming this way,
I suggest that you leave the area.'
Our reply was clear and firm:
'We will not leave, we are people's heroes.
We will face the enemy forces.'
When the enemy forces advanced
We showered them with bullets.

Kimathi's wife was the Secretary
Of the gallant fighting women's wing
Bren-gunned in their hideouts by the enemy.

You home guards are thieves and robbers
You always wait for the day of operation
To go to people's homes to maim and to loot.

What do you home guards fight for?
You fight for slavery
While we Mau Mau fight for this, our land
And Black people's freedom.

The child of the home guards, when he cries,
He is hushed: 'Stop crying,
Father will bring goods from patrol tonight.
He will bring us much meat tonight.'

5. In 1954 under the co-called Operation Anvil, the British Government arrested and
   detained more than 100,000 innocent Kenyans. The majority of these were taken to
   Manyani and Mackinnon Road detention camps.
6. Embakasi was a Special Branch centre during the Mau Mau struggle. All kinds of
   tortures against Kenyan patriots were perpetrated here. Ian Henderson was in
   charge of the centre.

When the Mau Mau child cries,
He is told to stop crying,
For the home guards will hear him
And come and capture him.

The greatest patriots of Kenya today
Are Kimathi and Mathenge,
Matenjagwo and Mbaria.

Line Up the Traitors

Who was there to witness
Our heroic deeds
When we attacked Eliud's[7] home guard camp?
Eliud ran and hid in the forest.

Heavy rain fell on our way to Eliud's camp
But with Major BatuBatu in command
We braved the rain
And arrived at the camp in time.

We made a stop at Kamugoiri
To plan for our strategy.
The major commanded:
'Surround the camp,
Eliminate every home guard
And release all prisoners.'

We caught the home guards by surprise,
We cut many down as they tried to escape,
Others dropped their guns and surrendered.
But Eliud managed to escape.

After releasing the prisoners,
Commander Kariba said:
'Line up all the traitors,
And shoot them one by one,
We have no time to waste.'

After eliminating the traitors,

7. Eliud was a colonial chief in Nyeri District during the war of National Liberation.

Commander Kariba again gave orders:
'Collect all the captured enemy's guns,
Burn down the camp and enemy's shops.'

Eliud, you and your home guard traitors
Know that we live in the forest
Fighting for our land
And freedom for African people,
We shall never never give up!

The Enemy Warplanes Came at Dawn

It was on the 10th day of June
The enemy warplanes came at dawn.
They surprised the guerrillas who were asleep,
The guerrillas ran for cover.
Ngai is great;
They were not discovered.

Chorus
Thai, Thai Thathaiya Ngai,
Ngai is great
We were not discovered.

After the planes had gone
Wambugu selected three guerrillas
To stand on guard against the enemy.

After the guards patrolled around
They suddenly rushed back to the base, saying:
'Evacuate the base immediately, the enemy forces are coming!'
We all left the base.

We left the base and headed for the mountains.
On our way to the mountains
The enemy planes circled over us.
We were bombed and bren-gunned,
For safety we hid in animal dens.

After the enemy planes had gone
Watoria asked Commander Gichuki
To call the guerrillas for prayers
To pray for the missing guerrilla guards.

After the prayers Watoria said to Commander Gichuki:
'We better go down the valley
To look for a place to sleep in
It is very late now
We cannot reach the next base.'

We were awakened at four on the morning of Friday.
Before finishing our breakfast
We were given orders to pack
And head west to the Headquarters.
When we arrived at the Headquarters
We met our comrades
We embraced one another with joy.

The Great Battle of Timau

Who was in Timau
When the children of Mumbi attacked
The airfield at 'Thundani's'?
We were fully prepared.
Thebeni fired the first shot
Then with the accuracy and rhythm of a guitar,
He fed the enemy with bullets.

Chorus
Listen to a great story
Of the Mau Mau guerrillas,
Who have roamed over valleys and hills
And seen a lot in their wanderings.

It was about four in the afternoon.
The Major stood up to cheer us up.
He said: 'Have no fear,
Abdullah will be in front.'

We were fully prepared
To storm 'Thundani's' home,
Though fenced with stone
And topped with broken glass.

Thundani came out thinking he would scare us.
But he ran back fast,
He and his wife and her friend.

Our Major then directed us:
'When you go in smash the cases
And search everything until you find the firearms.'

Later at Ngarariga forest
The fighters told him:
'We must not stay here,
It is unsafe and we will endanger ourselves.'

We moved down to Kanoru's estate,
But we were not safe there either.
We were harrassed daily by the colonial forces.

Because of the home guards' constant provocation
At Mbari ya Kiharu's
And mindful of hurting people in their homes,
Unwillingly, we fought back and beat them.

There was great rejoicing back
At the coffee estate
Because of our heroic deeds
Under our leader's guidance.

We Hoisted Our Liberation Flag

It was on a Tuesday evening
In a house down in the valley
The enemy decided to come up
To spy on the Gikuyu country.

Chorus
Be happy, be happy parents!
The trouble is over in Gikuyuland.

On our arrival in the valley
We hoisted our liberation flag.[8]
When the colonialist forces saw it
They took cover.

---

8. Commonly the Mau Mau guerrillas carried a red flag during their engagements with
the enemy forces, symbolizing their indomitability and patriotism.

Commander Kariba ordered boldly:
'Blow all whistles now!'
And after this signal was given
Our bullets were whistling everywhere.

Commander Kariba said again:
'We had better move from near people's homes
And fight in the banana valley.'

When we arrived near Ndungu's fig tree
The enemy was put to flight
By the sound of our sten guns.

When we actually reached Ndungu's fig tree
Rongu fired his machine gun
Flushing the remaining enemies from hiding.

Battle of Kayahwe River

Kayahwe is a very bad river,
Kayahwe is a very bad river,
Kayahwe is a very bad river –
That is where our heroes perished.

I will go mother, I will go,
I will go mother, I will go,
I will go mother, I will go,
I will go and see Kayahwe.

General Kago gets no sleep,
General Ihuura gets no sleep,
Our guerrillas get no sleep,
When they remember Kayahwe.

Battle of Tumutumu Hill

Friends, listen.
Hear this story about Tumutumu Hill
So that you may realize that Mwene-Nyaga is with us
And will never forsake us.

We had great fighters in our army:
Kagume and Ngecu and Kaburu;
While Baranja was at the trumpet
And Burunji was our secretary.

It was on a Wednesday towards noon,
We were in a village in the valley.
Our enemies climbed up the hill
In order to secretly observe our positions.

When it struck one in the afternoon
Baranja was sent further down the valley
Dressed like a peasant woman
In order to spy on the enemy.

He brought back important information:
That Kirimukuyu
Was heavily covered with colonial forces
While we had 400 guerrillas at Ngurumo
Whom the enemy wanted to attack.

However, victory was with us
Because Kongania, our woman contact,
Brought us an important message
And thus saved a thousand lives.

When it struck three o'clock
A thunderous noise was heard
From the top of the hill
And bren guns were firing from every direction;
We fought back bravely until the enemy ran in retreat.

Burunji gave his own life
To save the lives of his comrades:
He lit the fuse and threw a grenade
And their machine guns went dead.
Such a great victory for our guerrilla army!

Battle of Lukenya

While fighting in the forests,
Encamped in the coffee fields,
We young fighters planned our attack on Lukenya Prison.

When the discussion was over
And we had all agreed,
Our scouts were sent to investigate.

They went and returned,
Giving us a report:
We should prepare ourselves for the attack.

We began our journey toward Lukenya
Keeping well-hidden all the way,

When we arrived our fighters lay down;
We opened fire and killed two guards.

The black people imprisoned were crying for help,
Saying: 'Oh, our people, open the doors for us!'

After fighting and releasing the prisoners,
We prayed to Ngai in us
So that he might assist us to return safely.

All black people of Nairobi were happy
Congratulating us for our brave deeds.

Battle of Kaaruthi Valley

One day about 3 o'clock
In the valley at Kaaruthi
We were planning our strategy
After learning that we were closely covered.

We hoisted our flag
And we began to move.
When the enemy forces saw this,
They were most frightened.

When the guerrillas confronted the enemy
Parents were very much worried
Thinking that the enemy would exterminate our entire unit.

An elderly woman contact
Brought us information.
Tearfully she said:

'My children you must flee
Danger surrounds you.'

We comforted her and explained;
'When we guerrillas fight, their bullets
Fly way above us in the trees.
We are fully prepared.'
Suddenly the bullets were flying
Across the banana fields.

The masses were overjoyed
When we hoisted our flag in a victory
Loud ululations and thunderous applause
Were heard, up and down, Rui-Ruiru.[9]

At four many whites came at Rui-Ruiru
Hoping to witness the extermination
Of our guerrilla unit
They left in disappointment.

We had laid in ambush near the Mugumo tree.
Rongu fired his machine gun.
The whistles went off,
The battle was on.

We'd fire our Gatua-Uhoro[10]
They'd all drop down in fear.
When they fired their bazooka
We all took cover.

Many colonialist forces were there
Brought from Nanyuki
Others from Tumutumu
And yet more from Karatina.

Then Commander Kariba said:
'Concentrate on white soldiers,
Leave the Black puppets for the time being
We will deal with them later.'

When the guerrillas were crossing Ruthagati
Ruhiu was the Major, the Commander in Charge,

9. A river called Rui-Ruiru in Nyeri.
10. See Appendix.

And the leader of the guerrilla unit.

When we arrived at Kiangi
We learned that the enemy was in ambush.
From their rear we caught them by surprise
They all scattered and ran.

Most of the enemy soldiers ran
Heading for Kiamacimbi.
They were using radio desperately
Calling Nanyuki for reinforcements.
But in vain, we shall surely win!

At Mombasa port, as they leave our land
The whites will weep.
They will shed bitter tears, saying:
'We have been forced to leave Kenya
A land of milk and honey.'

And the traitors who collaborated
With our enemies will be most ashamed
To see that those they used to insult and torture
Will then be the rulers of Kenya.

Appendix: The Development of New Words and Concepts

We learn from the songs that Mau Mau was referring to a new society. Many words were new concepts and terms used to represent the birth of a new nation. They also reflected qualitative changes in our anti-colonial culture. For example:

Muingi	Masses
Kirindi	Masses
Wiyathi	Independence
Uiguano wa andu a Kenya	Unity of the Kenyan people
Mbara ya wiyathi	War of independence
Mbara ya Muingi	People's war
Ngwatanirwo ya Muingi	Solidarity of the masses
Wendo wa bururi witu	Patriotism
Andu aitu	Our compatriots/our people
Itugi cia bururi	Patriotic 'servants' of the people
Muma wa Uiguano	The oath of unity by which individuals were initiated into the Movement
Muhimu (Swahili)	A cover word for the Movement meaning 'most important.'

Other terms symbolized the heroism and patriotism of our Mau Mau guerrilla army. These concepts were an echo of the militant spirit of our fighting forces, an echo of the inexhaustible determination of the Mau Mau guerrillas to liberate our Motherland from the foreign occupiers:

Ihii cia Mutitu	Mau Mau guerrillas
Ihii cia Mbuci	Mau Mau guerrillas
Itungati	Fighters
Mirani	Guerrillas
Nyumba iitu	Our comrades/our compatriots
Njamba cia ruriri	Heroes of the nation
Njamba cia Muingi	People's heroes
Njamba cia bururi	Heroes of the country
Mbuci	Mau Mau guerrilla's base
Mbutu	Battalion

113

Muma wa Batuni   The platoon oath given only to those
patriots who had been selected by the
Mau Mau Central Committee to join the
guerrilla army.

Further terms were coined which arose in connection with the rise of new
cultural consciousness among the masses. They also represented and symbolized a whole chain of Mau Mau heroism and events:

Gatua-Uhoro	Name of the gun manufactured by Mau Mau guerrillas. Literally means 'the decider'.
Makara	Ammunition. Literally, 'charcoal'.
Muti	Rifle. Literally, a 'stick'.
Kamuti	Hand gun or pistol. Literally, a 'small stick'.
Njirungi	Ammunition.
Bebeta	Machine gun, bren gun or sten gun.
Mucinga wa nyoni	Shot-gun.
Kamwaki	Same as *Kamuti* above.
Gutharenda	To surrender or to collaborate with the enemy.
Komerera (verb)	To hide from the enemy; to join the Mau Mau army in the forest.

Along with these, the following class terms were also developed:

Hinga	Person who betrays others. The word commonly referred to the loyalist traitors and African elite who had sold out to the British enemy during the struggle. Literally, the word means a 'hypocrite'.
Eririri	Those who sided with the enemy during the resistance. This group of traitors committed untold crimes against Kenyans during the war. They were used by the British colonialists as a terrorist army. They enriched themselves through looting and plundering everything they could lay their hands on. This group went on to assume the role of a comprador bourgeoisie class. Literally, the term means 'those individuals who solely think of their stomachs'.
Thaka	The petty bourgeoisie who betrayed the people and who joined the enemy forces during the Mau Mau war of national independence.
Thata cia bururi	Commonly used to refer to traitors during the struggle; particularly it

	referred to the home guard traitors. Literally, means the 'barren of the land'.
Tai-tai	Petty-bourgeois fifth columnists during the Mau Mau war. Most of these traitors were operating in Nairobi. Literally, it meant 'those who wore ties – i.e. the elite.
Gakonia	A hooded and masked individual who acted as a British colonial agent during the national struggle. He was used to identify members and cadres of the Mau Mau Movement. Literally, the word refers to the sisal or hessian sacking material used for the hood.
Kamatimu	Popular name for the home guard traitors. Literally, it means 'a spear bearer'.
Gatimu or *Gatheci*	Same as *Kamatimu* above.
Thambara	African informer during the struggle. Literally, a 'leech'.
Thuthi	A colonial government agent or a spy during the Mau Mau war. Literally, a 'weevil' or 'worm'.
Thuiya	Those individuals who had not taken the oath. They were not harmful to the Movement, but they were not supposed to know the secrets of the Movement. Literally, the word means a 'flea'.
Thu cia Bururi	Traitors to the land, or the enemy of the country.
Kuhunga Mahuri	To interrogate or screen.
Muhungi wa Mahuri	Police interrogator.
Athungu airu	African elites who sided with the British colonialists against Mau Mau. Normally referred to individuals like Tom Mbotela, Ofafa and big colonial chiefs like Waruhiu, Nderi, etc. Literally, 'black-skinned Europeans'.
Maguru Mairu	Black mercenaries in the colonial police force. Literally, it means 'black legs' after the customary black strapping material used as stockings.
Gicakuri	Mercenary soldier. Literally, a 'pitchfork'.
Warurungana	Commonly used for the paramilitary police composed of mercenaries from

	Northern Kenya,
Thukumu	Imperialism. It can also refer to an imperialist or imperialists.
Thukumu ya Ngeretha	British imperialism.
Ukoroni	Colonialism.
Mukoroni	A colonialist.
Ukoroni wa Ngeretha	British colonialism.
Kemerera (noun)	Mau Mau deserters and rejects who escaped to avoid military and political discipline. They became notorious for terrorizing peasants and robbing them at night posing as Mau Mau guerrillas. They thus did considerable damage to the Movement's work among the general population and may have helped isolate the guerrillas from their main supporters. The Mau Mau War Council ordered them eliminated summarily whenever they were caught and General Kago is reputed to have carried out a special campaign aimed at this 'burglar brigade'.

These class terms were used to refer to, and identify, the enemy of the Movement. Popular words such as *Kimendero* (the one who crushes or eliminates) and *John wa Mahuri* (a name coined by the people to refer to a particular home guard in Murang'a District) referred to the individual home guard traitors who were well known in Central Kenya for terrorizing and murdering the unarmed population during the struggle. These individuals were so infamous that people were known to run for their lives when they appeared on the scene.